BEAUTIFUL
BODY
BEAUTIFUL
SKIN

BEAUTIFUL BODY
BEAUTIFUL SKIN

Norma Knox

PIATKUS

First published in 1990 by
Judy Piatkus (Publishers) Ltd of
5 Windmill Street, London W1P 1HF

Reprinted in 1993

**The moral right of the author
has been asserted**

*A catalogue record for this book is available
from the British Library*

ISBN 0–7499–1046–1

Designed by Paul Saunders
Illustrated by Caroline Bays
Cover design by Jerry Goldie
Cover photograph courtesy of Clarins Paris

Typeset in 11/13 Linotron Plantin Light by
Phoenix Photosetting, Chatham
Printed and bound in Great Britain at
The Bath Press, Bath, Avon

The author and publishers would like to thank the following companies for supplying
cosmetics as featured in the line illustrations: Max Factor; Secret Garden; Boots 2000;
Aapri; Buf-puf. The author and publishers would also like to thank the following
companies for kindly supplying colour photographs: Barbara Daly's Colourings
(pp 144–5, photographer Robert Mackintosh; pictures taken from 'Face to Face' video
available from The Body Shop); Lil-lets (p 33); Harley Medical Group (p 129); Nivea
Sun (p 49); Biotherm (p 48); Innoxa (p 128); Lancôme (p 32).

ACKNOWLEDGEMENTS

I am not a scientist, dermatologist or beauty therapist, so I needed help with much of this book. I'm grateful to all the experts who gave me information, time and patiently corrected my copy when necessary.

I'd like to say a special thanks to: Pat Richardson, journalist and friend (for extra research and always being willing to discuss the subject); David A Fenton, Senior Registrar, Dowling Skin Unit, St. Thomas' Hospital, London (for simplifying the difficult and checking so many words); John Hawk, Head of Photobiology, St. Thomas' Hospital; Diane Miles, pharmacist and marketing manager for Christian Dior; Dr Gordon Russell, Ciba Geigy; Eve Taylor, beauty therapist, aromatherapist and friend; Marylyn Ennever, press secretary, British Association of Electrolysists; Leonard Mervyn of Healthcrafts Ltd; all the health and beauty PRs who've helped me on this book and in the past.

I would also like to thank Bryce Knox, my husband, who fed, watered and wined me, corrected my spelling and was endlessly tolerant as I developed a new enthusiasm with each chapter.

The more I delved into skin, the less I felt I knew about it. Special thanks to the dermatologist who, as I wailed about my ignorance, said 'Join the club!'

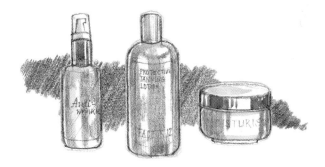

Note

Before going on any diet, or doing any exercises mentioned in this book, do check with your doctor if you have any doubts about your state of health.

CONTENTS

INTRODUCTION

First of all let me emphasise that skin care is for *everyone* – men, women and children. The earliest possible start will help your skin to work better for you for much longer, but it's never too late to make improvements. Wanting a smooth, blemish-free skin is not just a matter of vanity. Trouble with your skin almost invariably means something is amiss with your body – hence the title of this book, *Beautiful Body, Beautiful Skin*.

While you are looking after your skin, you will be doing good things for your body and also working on that crucial relationship between mind and body. Your whole self has to be in reasonable order for your skin to look its best. As the owner of an always highly reactive skin, I'm a prime example of the mind/body relationship; I've been living with a nasty patch of adult acne on my chin from the moment I agreed to write this book and add more work to an already hectic life. Stress is the current buzz-word that's blamed for everything, but it certainly jostles with the sun as skin enemy number one.

While some of us (including me) make a fuss about the odd outbreak of spots or some newly observed signs of age in the mirror, it's important to remember that there are people – many of them – who suffer a lifetime of distressing, disfiguring and life-crippling skin defects through no fault of their own. Hopefully, there's help in these pages for everyone, whatever their age, sex or state of skin. But there is no-one quite like you. I can give you guidelines on diet, exercise and skin care that should help you to look better in every way, but a product or routine that's perfect for some people may not work for you. So listen to *your* body, learn to read its likes and dislikes and work with it whenever you can.

I've added this introduction after completing the final chapter, so it's time to start practising what I preach, putting my whole self in order and getting my skin on an even keel once more. Won't you join me?

Norma Knox
Blackheath, September 1989

CHAPTER ONE

GET TO KNOW YOUR SKIN

In an ideal world, most of us would call a halt to skin development somewhere in late childhood. This way we'd avoid the coarsening, oiliness and eruptions of puberty and the progressive lines, sags and blotches of age. And most men would surely choose another way to spend something like the 3,500 hours of their lives now devoted to taking the bristles off their faces. But before you moan about your own particular skin chores or problems . . . STOP . . . and consider what your skin does for you and your body.

WHAT IS SKIN?

Your skin is a multi-layered, constantly renewing structure consisting of three distinct regions all closely connected and working together. It is the largest organ of the body. The average adult's skin covers about 2 square metres and weighs 2½ to 3½ kilos, and apart from the brain is the most complex and hard-working one. Unlike other organs that are covered, protected and cosseted at a constant temperature, it's out there up front acting as your first line of defence against every enemy in the environment from bacteria to bad weather and a brush with a dangerous object.

As well as holding you neatly in place with the minimum restriction, it prevents your body from dehydrating (one of the reasons severe burns are so dangerous), regulates body temperature, does a first-class waste disposal job, warns you of potential pain and telegraphs pleasure from the enjoyable touches in life (like massage, a kiss, a caress).

The surface of the hard protective top layer (actually several interwoven layers) is constantly wearing away and is just as constantly being replaced. On the whole, skin maintains and repairs itself very effectively *and* it does all these jobs for your entire lifetime. Certainly some skins have a longer beautiful life than others – and for beautiful read youthful – and this has much to do with genetics. Someone in your family has passed on the right or wrong genes.

But you can help your hereditary characteristics both from inside and outside. A healthy lifestyle with sensible eating and drinking habits, regular exercise and relaxation, stress and anxiety control whenever possible and protection from your environment can all help your skin to function well and stay in optimum condition. There's much more to skin than what you see, so let's go beyond the surface.

BEYOND THE SURFACE

In the beauty side of the skin business there are some wonderful 'did you know?' one-liners like 'In the time it takes you to travel from the bottom to the top of an underground escalator you will have inhaled all the dead skin cells from one human being' and 'Ninety per cent of household dust is made up of dead skin cells.' To the first I'd say, 'How long is an escalator and are we in a rush hour?' And to the second, 'Not if, like mine, your household includes a couple of golf fanatics who deposit half a pound of mud inside the front door after a game, plus a very hairy cat who'll fill the vacuum bag inside a week.' But it is certainly true that, in a far less spectacular way than snakes, we are continuously throwing off our old skin and just as continuously coming up with a new one.

While our immediate concern is usually with what faces us in the mirror, the skin you see is only the tip of the iceberg or, to put it more correctly, a horny layer of dead, old, keratinised cells that are similar in substance to horses' hooves, cows' horns and human hair and nails. Let's take a deeper look at the skin and its three regions: the outermost layer (epidermis), the true skin (dermis) and the lower layer (hypodermis).

The Epidermis
The epidermis varies in thickness – it's thinner on your eyelids than on the rest of your face and thicker on the soles of the feet and palms of the hands than on the rest of the body. Thick or thin, the epidermis consists of layers of cells that are continuously dividing in the lower part (the basal layer) and moving up to the surface where they fall or are rubbed off. On their journey upwards and outwards they flatten and die, and chemical changes

take place which transform them into a hard, durable protein called keratin on the outermost part of the skin. This horny layer, known as the *stratum corneum*, is in fact constructed of many overlapping layers rather like a tiled roof. If the roof is well-maintained, the skin will refract light and look smooth and beautiful. But of course, life isn't like that. Some of the tiles turn up at the edges, and slip but don't fall immediately.

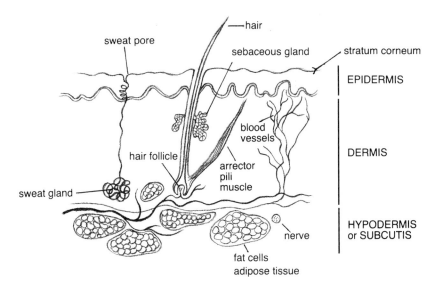

Beneath the surface of the skin

This is where skin beauty care comes into its own. Exfoliators speed the path of dead skin cells and stimulate the basal layer to fresh cell production. The transit time of cells from birth in the basal layer to the surface of your skin is about 3–4 weeks and by an ingenious control system new cells are manufactured very precisely in number to match those lost, so there's no danger of skin wearing out. The system does slow with age – cuts take longer to heal and older skin won't look as fresh as a young person's.

Moisturisers have the effect of supplementing your own natural moisturising system which comes from the secretions of the sweat and sebaceous glands and water released by epidermal cells as they complete their lifespan. Sebum, sweat and evaporating moisture mix to form a protective, slightly acidic emulsion on the skin's surface. More seriously your life depends on this two-way 'waterproof' layer. It quite literally stops you getting soaked to the bone when it rains and helps to protect your body from almost everything life throws at it. Working the other way, it prevents potentially fatal dehydration – without a horny protective layer we'd be dead in a matter of hours.

Down in the basal layer are the melanocytes – the melanin producing cells responsible for skin pigmentation. The distribution and quality of these cells play a major role in the colour of our skin. Melanin's ability to absorb ultra-violet light gives our bodies a degree of natural sunscreening. Exposure to sunlight stimulates melanin production and alters the pattern of distribution, so that less ultra-violet light reaches the lower layers of your skin.

The Dermis

The dermis or true skin fits neatly and closely on the underside of the epidermis rather like a child's jigsaw puzzle, and this is where much of the making and marring of your skin takes place. The dermis is situated beyond the reach of skin care products, although *skin care* can help prolong its active, beautiful life. While the dermis contains various types of cell, it is the fibroblasts that manufacture the network of interlacing bundles of fibrous tissues – collagen and elastin – that prop up the epidermis and are so vital to the youthful look of skin. When these fibres harden and bunch up, the elastic qualities of the skin weaken, so it no longer snaps back smoothly into place or fits so neatly after any movement of the skin (in fact it works, or doesn't work, just like a piece of elastic – this is one of the reasons why lines are more obvious where there is much muscle or joint movement, for instance around the eyes or elbows).

While medical research with fibroblasts suggests these cells possess their own biological time clock which allows them to work a certain and very set number of times – suggesting that the ageing factor is part of your genetic programming – things like stringent dieting, excessive exposure to the sun or severe illness can deplete the water content of this layer, diminishing the efficiency of the connective tissue and leading to premature lines, wrinkles and sagging skin. On the optimistic side of skin health, this is the area that benefits most from a healthy, well-balanced lifestyle.

The dermis is rich in blood vessels and lymphatic channels which nourish and oxygenate your skin and eliminate waste products. This area contains the sweat glands and ducts, the hair follicles with their accompanying sebaceous glands and the *arrector pili* muscles. These are the involuntary muscles which give you goose pimples and make your hair stand on end when you're cold, thrilled or frightened. Take a look at the family pet or wild birds in the garden during cold weather and you'll see their fur or feathers fluffed up to trap air around the skin to form an insulating layer. While we humans now lack sufficient hair to keep us warm, the prehistoric reaction continues and the muscle action alone goes some way towards raising body temperature in cold conditions.

Finally, the dermis contains the nerve endings that register the good and bad touches in life – tell us whether we're hot, cold, being tickled, caressed, pinched or punched.

The Hypodermis

The hypodermis (also known as the *subcutis*) is the deepest layer of skin and serves to 'featherbed' the body. Composed mainly of fat cells stored in connective tissue, it protects the blood, lymph and nerve tracts in the dermis, cushions the body from blows and keeps it warm. Thin people feel the cold more than fat ones and consequently most men feel it more than most women who tend to have more insulating fat in their bodies. This fatty layer, or to give it its more pleasing name, adipose tissue, varies in thickness from one area of the body to another. It's thin on the bridge of the nose, the breastbone and spine, and thick on the buttocks. Women who are designed to be rounded to protect their unborn babies, have a different fat distribution from men.

The hypodermis serves as an energy depot on which the body can draw when in need. This can be done involuntarily in the case of serious illness or starvation or voluntarily during crash diets. Athletes will burn off much of this layer during long, regular exercise sessions and women athletes tend to lose the 'female fat' distribution.

The hypodermis also plays an important role in separating the dermis from the muscles and underlying structure of the body, so the skin moves freely as our bodies go into action.

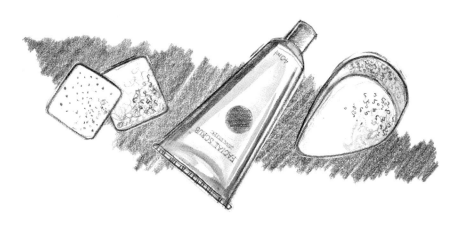

DETERMINING YOUR SKIN TYPE

While the state of your skin, good or bad, has much to do with heredity, hormones and your lifestyle, keeping it clean and protected plays a very important part in its surface condition and long-lasting looks. The human body is made up of about seventy per cent water, and fifteen per cent or more of this is in the dermis. The outermost layer of your skin – the part you see and skin care and beauty products work on – depends for its youthful looks and resilience on a constant supply of water from the lower layers and its ability to retain that water without losing too much through evaporation. Also up there on the surface, sebum (the fatty secretion of the sebaceous glands), sweat and evaporating water mingle to form a slightly acidic, protective emulsion called the hydro-lipidic film which in turn helps to prevent excessive evaporation of water. It's a perfect irrigation system when all is working well, but so much can upset it.

Even a normal skin can dry out if it spends most of its days stuck in the dry atmosphere of many air-conditioned buildings or goes through a long winter of temperature changes from over-enthusiastic central heating indoors to icy cold and skin-stripping winds outside. All the hormonal changing conditions such as periods, pregnancy, menopause, and even the Pill, can throw out the natural balance of your skin. Other culprits might be air travel, a holiday in the sun, drastic dieting and over-harsh or poor cleansing processes. Illness, even a relatively minor one that's treated with over-the-counter medicaments, can change your skin's behaviour.

Sebum output and the skin's natural moisture content diminish as we grow older. And a down period at any time in your life when you're short of sleep, eating irregularly or living with negative stress can play havoc with your skin.

Nothing remains static on the skin front and you may be weary of hearing talk of dry, oily or combination skin when yours seems to vary from day to day, and certainly from season to season. But you really do have a basic type, which will naturally move to drier, wherever it starts, as the years go by. Skin care companies spend a fortune researching ingredients that will help counteract natural imbalances and adverse conditions, so when you're buying products, aim for the category formulated for your skin's usual behaviour, but keep a careful check for any changes.

NORMAL SKIN

Normal skin is finely textured, lively-looking, and smooth to the touch. It doesn't shine, dry up, flake or develop spots. You see it all the time on children – but it's not so common in adults. While the most obvious characteristic of a normal skin is the absence of problems, it's usually short-lived and will have a tendency to dryness quite early in life. It needs careful treatment, close monitoring and good health and beauty routines.

DRY SKIN

Dry skin looks fine, close textured and attractive when young and well-cared for, but it can flake, chap, feel tight, and be fragile and is certainly a candidate for premature surface lines unless it's well lubricated and protected from exposure to weather extremes and dry atmospheres and conditions. It's usually the one with few puberty problems and the much envied 'English Rose' complexion usually falls into this category. This skin type thrives in British weather conditions but should not be out in the sun without wearing a sun block, and central heating can drain it. Invest in a humidifier in centrally heated homes or at least keep pots of water in rooms to keep up the humidity. Don't face the day without wearing a moisturiser and go for rich, water-in-oil creams at night. Take special care of the eye area, which is always drier.

SENSITIVE SKIN

Sensitive skins take all the problems of dry skins a few stages further. This skin can be beautiful, almost translucent at its best, but it's likely to suffer at a puff of wind, develop redness and small surface veins, and be allergic to certain ingredients in products, and it's another early ager. This skin often belongs to people who suffer from hay fever, asthma, or other allergies. Stay away from extremes of weather and the sun as much as possible. Keep centrally heated and air conditioned rooms humidified and use the gentlest touch, and the kindest products – those specifically formulated for sensitive skins and without perfume or any ingredients that are likely to cause allergic reactions. It's wise to buy products that list ingredients, so it's easy to check if there's something your skin doesn't agree with.

OILY SKIN

At puberty the male hormones that make a boy a man also increase the amount of sebum produced. But men produce small quantities of female hormones and vice versa so it's oil time for more or less everyone as a teen-ager. No-one who has a greasy skin needs to have it described. Constant shine, enlarged openings where sebum pours out, possibly a regular tussle with blackheads and blemishes and – for the female – make-up that melts away almost as soon as it's applied. On the plus side, the oil is a natural moisture retainer and, with care, this skin looks younger longer. When the oiliness continues into the twenties and beyond, it often accompanies Mediterranean looks – dark hair and eyes, an olive skin which, when protected, can take the sun and look super.

While this type of skin is more resilient than drier ones, don't be lulled into a false sense of security and neglect it or treat it with harsh cleansers that may strip the oil and could encourage flaking and extra oil production to compensate. From the twenties onwards, take care of the eyes and neck which can fall into the dry skin category even when the rest of your face is oily.

COMBINATION SKIN

Combination skin is the type most of us live with from post puberty to middle age. The central area of everyone's head and body contains more sebaceous glands than the outskirts, and on the face the oilier area can include chin, nose and forehead – the much talked of T-zone – which will be coarser textured than the rest of your face.

If you're not certain whether you fall into this category, you can always try the tissue test: cleanse your face, leave it naked of products for half an hour, then lay an open white tissue over it. Gently press the tissue against the contours of your face with your fingers. Wherever there's grease, the tissue will be grey. Combination skin needs combination care, so that each area gets the right treatment to maintain its correct oil/moisture balance. Eyes, cheeks and neck can dry up while the central patch stays oily, so always watch them carefully.

While extreme skin conditions or lack of oil and/or moisture will be obvious, it's sometimes difficult to decide for yourself your skin's exact category. Indeed, certain skins can appear to be oily, but are in fact lacking in moisture. This can happen through illness, some crazy crash dieting, constant exposure to weather extremes and air conditioning or after excessive use of diuretics and laxatives. It's a very good idea to have a regular professional facial, certainly an occasional one, as a beauty therapist will be able to pinpoint your needs. Some have a skin scanner which uses UV light to detect conditions which are barely visible even to the professional's naked eye.

SKIN TEST

Use the guide opposite to help you to identify your skin type from the way it looks, feels and behaves, so you can give it the right type of external treatment. When it's clean and free of make-up and moisturiser for at least an hour (and preferably during the afternoon when it's well into its day behaviour), move your mirror to a good light near a large window with you facing outwards and carry out your examination. Keep a note of your findings and remember to re-check from time to time to keep up with any alterations due to different seasons, the passing years, trouble spots in your life, major hormonal changes, holidays, and so on.

Combination skin

Combination skin looks and behaves like more than one skin type. If you don't fit into a category note the characteristics by ticking the relevant 'look and behaviour' items so you can treat the different areas according to type. Many skin houses are labelling their products for normal/oily skins, normal/dry skins, etc, which is helpful as few faces have an even oil output overall.

SPECIAL CASES

For countless thousands of years most people were born, lived and died a matter of a few miles from where their ancestors had been born, lived and died, and skins naturally evolved to cope with the conditions and climates of particular parts of the world. Soft, pale 'Irish' skin was perfectly suited to the damp mists and moderate temperatures of that country; and Asian and African skins to high temperatures, humidity and baking sun. But transportation and emigration, which has been taking place for three hundred years or so and has greatly increased in the present century, have now placed pale skins in baking climates and dark skins in cold ones. Adapting to life in climates they were not 'made' for can cause difficulties.

'Irish' or Celtic skin

Pale, delicate skin often accompanying very dark or reddish hair is frequently found in people of Irish and Scottish descent. It is smooth and blemish-free, the stuff that poems are penned to in its prime. It often becomes translucent and beautiful in old age, but this softness, lack of colour (and often oil) can bring problems with early loss of elasticity, premature wrinkling, and a tendency to react irritably to beauty treatments like waxing and electrolysis. It can also collapse under the

How your skin will look

If it is **normal**:
- even texture
- minimal lines
- no shine
- lively, bright tone

If it is **sensitive and/or dehydrated**:
- very fine texture
- premature very fine lines

If it is **oily**:
- coarse texture
- shine
- possible blemishes

If it is **dry**:
- fine texture
- fine surface lines
- dryness, flakiness
- it looks good when young and nothing upsets it.

- skin looks stretched
- flaking/blotching/irritated areas

- few, if any, lines (deeper ones round mobile areas – eyes, mouth – if you're older)

How your skin behaves

If it is **normal** it:
- is relatively trouble free
- will feel supple
- rarely has a spot, a blemish

If it's **dry** it:
- behaves badly in weather extremes
- can't get enough moisturiser

If it's **sensitive** it will be:
- terribly touchy
- taut and papery to touch
- inclined to redness, surface veins

If it's **oily** it will:
- be quite resilient
- soak up cosmetics, particularly in warm weather
- often look and feel grubby by the afternoon

- takes most treatment and make-up beautifully

- sometimes feels rough and 'chapped'
- is unpredictable

- upset by many things, from temperature extremes to some beauty treatments and products

- be prone to blemishes, particularly if you are tense, unwell or around menstruation time

strain of pregnancy, leaving stretch marks and loss of elasticity on the abdominal area.

Emigration in the past means these skins are often placed in hot parts of the States and Australia where strong sun will encourage the early ageing tendency and can bring major skin problems. Heat and increased surface circulation can lead to obvious veins on the surface of this soft skin. 'Irish' skin needs a gentle touch and plenty of protection from extreme weather conditions, central heating or air conditioning . . . and moisturising at all times.

Oriental skin

The sebum output of Oriental skin can be as variable as that of Caucasian skins, but it is genetically stronger and more resilient, so ageing comes later . . . very late if it's sheltered from hot sun. This is usually a fine, smooth, even-toned skin and the facial structure is markedly less angular than the European – with flat cheekbones and small nose – which can mean less character lines around mouth and eyes. Although this skin can usually cope with hot sun, it lacks the red tones of tanned Caucasian skins and can become muddy-looking and suffer from pigmentation patching when exposed to the rays.

Asian skin

A strong skin that basically takes a lot of wear and tear without showing signs of age. In Asia it easily acclimatises to the heat and rainy seasons, but in Britain and northern European countries it can become very dry and suffer from pigmentation problems on cheeks, nose and forehead from a combination of climate changes, central heating and strip lighting. Mrs Puri of Shahnaz Herbal in London finds 'lack of time' is a beauty problem for her Asian and British clients. 'In India women are more beauty orientated. They have massage, use oils and Ayurvedic medicine (an ancient Hindu health system which makes use of the powers of nature, special diets, massage with herbal oils and meditation for the maintenance of health, energy and youthful looks). Ordinary working girls will spend money on treatments for beauty, body and soul . . . even very poor women care about their looks, use oils and will, for instance, take a piece of charcoal from the fire and use it to remove every trace of hair from their legs.'

Afro-Caribbean skin. . .

The description 'black skin' can cover the spectrum from ivory to deep jet (there are thirty-four to thirty-eight recognised shades of black skin), but generally black skin has larger pigment granules than Caucasian and thus has a greater natural protection against ageing and damaging UV rays. Black skins have a higher oil secretion than Caucasian skins, which is also anti-ageing, but can bring possible texture and eruption troubles from time to time.

The continual shedding of dead skin cells which lack colour and don't show up too much on a white skin can be very obvious on black skins and rich emollients are essential to prevent an ashy tone, particularly in winter in northern climates where weather conditions and central heating accelerate the problem.

Uneven pigmentation may be a problem. Basically this means that there are many skin tones on one face. Skin lighteners may sometimes be used on small, darker patches, but this should only be done after taking expert advice and using special products that contain less than two per cent hydroquinone which is a strong lightening agent and should be used with caution. Even quite minor damage to black skin – a bad mosquito bite or a small cut – can heal leaving darker or lighter patches of skin. Vitiligo which again may be hardly noticeable on many white skins can be very obvious on dark skin. Camouflage cosmetics can be a great help where there are any pigmentation problems.

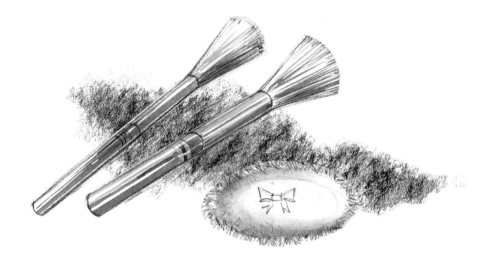

CHAPTER TWO

*C*LEANSING AND MOISTURISING

Even when you spend a relaxed day by the sea or in the country, by evening your face will be grubby, so just think what it's like if you pass a stressful day in a dirty town wearing full make-up. Your skin will be covered with an unpleasant mixture of grease and dirt, which, if left *in situ*, can become the ideal breeding ground for bacteria.

Now consider what comes off your face when you cleanse. The skin's a bit of a dustbin for the body with waste products constantly being eliminated on its surface together with oil and water. Add ready-to-fall dead surface cells, stale make-up and anything that's floating around in your particular environment and you'll understand the need for regular, thorough cleansing. It will make your face look brighter, fresher, and younger and your skin will be far more ready to accommodate anything you're going to put on it from sunscreens and moisturiser to fresh make-up. That doesn't mean going over the top. While it's very necessary to have a thorough cleanse at night to eliminate the day's grime and a freshening cleanse in the morning, leave your face to follow its own processes in between times. Constant clean-ups are unnecessary and time wasting, and could do more harm than good.

COMING CLEAN

Are you bewildered by cleanser choice – all those shelves full of super-fatted soaps, cleansing bars, soap substitutes, foaming facial liquids, lotions, gels, wash creams, creamy lotions and cream cleansers? And to add to the confusion there are astringents, skin toners, tonics, fresheners and all the extras – facial scrubs, masks, exfoliating creams, buff pads and sponges, loofah discs, complexion brushes, and clarifying lotions. What's wrong with a good old bar of soap, a flannel and some water, you might well ask?

SOAP AND WATER

Let's start with the flannel. A spotlessly clean, dry flannel (preferably white, so it can be boil washed) rubbed gently over your face makes a first class exfoliator – just see the 'dirt' that comes off what you thought was your clean face. If you use one for rinsing, again it should be boil washed after each use or it can become another cosy home for bacteria.

Soap is a very efficient cleanser, made from fats and caustic alkalis, that bite through dirt and grease. The trouble with ordinary soap is that it can work too thoroughly and upset the skin's natural acid balance and strip it of oil. Also, it doesn't work too well on oil-based make-ups which are just moved around by soap and water washing and the pigment content that doesn't come off on the towel will simply remain in a sludge on your face.

Manufacturers, aware of the demand for 'soap' and water washing for faces, have come up with super fatted, acid balanced cleansing bars which are kinder to skins. Water never was the harmful part of the soap and water formula and if you don't feel clean or wide awake if you haven't wet your face, there is also a host of rinse-away wash gels, lotions and creams (designed to remove make-up) now on the market, and many traditional cleansing creams and lotions now offer a wash-away option as an alternative to removal with cotton wool or tissues.

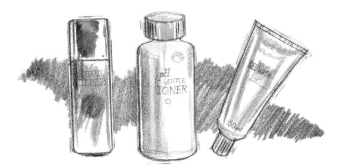

CLEANSERS

However luxurious and expensive the individual ingredients, most cleansing products that are designed to remove oil-based cosmetics are formulated in the same basic way. They include oil to break down the oil-soluble dirt and make-up and detergent-type products to emulsify the oil impurities and get the whole lot moving off your face. The oil/detergent ratio varies according to the skin type it's made for, with higher oil content for drier skins and a higher detergent content for oily ones. If you're still searching for a cleanser you like, read the labels and match your skin type. Judge by results. The right cleanser is one that leaves your skin looking clean and feeling comfortable.

How much should you pay for a cleanser? Again, the price is right if it suits your skin. Generally speaking, you will need less of an expensive cleanser to do an efficient job, so overall it won't cost so much more than a cheaper one. It's also worth remembering that cleansing is a very transient treatment; the product will be on your face for no more than a minute. Only the most sensitive skins will suffer for any length of time from using the 'wrong' cleanser.

Cleansers are formulated to remove make-up by dissolving it. Simply allow the product time to act, then wipe or wash it away – there's no need to

---

Make your own make-up remover pads

These 'professional' cleansing pads are much more efficient for face cleaning than tissues or tiny balls of cotton wool. Make enough for three or four days and store them, flat, in a plastic bag in the fridge.

1. From a roll of inexpensive surgical cotton wool, cut about six squares each measuring roughly six inches or 15cm on all sides.

2. Dip each square in clean, cold water, then squeeze out until barely damp.

3. Hold one corner and peel off layers – you'll get two or three pads from each square. Any small leftovers can be used to take off eye or lip make-up.

4. Fold the square you're going to use in half, then fold again in quarters. Hold it across the front of your middle two fingers, tucking the points between first and fourth fingers.

5. Change the fold of the pad frequently as you cleanse and massage your face and it will give you eight clean surfaces. If you use a lot of make-up, you may need two pads for a thorough cleanse. Then use another pad sprinkled with skin toner or freshener to wipe over the face after cleansing.

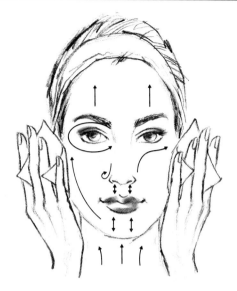

Remove make-up with professional strokes

First remove lip and eye make-up, then apply cleanser over your neck and face. With your cleansing square (or you can have one in each hand, so you do both sides of your face together) make the following moves.

1. Sweep upwards from neck to chin and make several sweeps moving from one side of the neck to the other.

2. Move up side of nose and across cheekbone towards ear.

3. Move up jawline from chin to ear.

4. Up forehead from brow to hairline working across from one side to the other.

5. Down nose and around nostrils working in little circles around them.

6. Up and down between chin and mouth and

7. Between upper lip and nose.

8. Finally sweep very lightly around eye from under inner brow across to outer edge of eye and under eye to nose.

rub or scrub at your skin. You can use cream or lotion cleansing sessions to give your face a stimulating massage.

TONERS

Astringents, toners (they may be called tonics) and fresheners are the various names given to the liquid toning products that provide the second step in completely removing make-up. The increase in water-rinsable cleansers has perhaps made them less essential, but they do have an important place in any good cleansing routine. The role of any toning product is to remove all traces of cleanser and dirt residue, gently stimulate surface circulation and help restore the skin's acid balance.

Astringents are the strongest, formulated for oily skins. But their once high alcohol content has increasingly given way to gentler ingredients as it became obvious that a naturally oily skin responds to over-harsh removal of excess oil with excess production. Indeed, most skin care houses are switching to gentle ingredients for all types of skin, so again be guided by the label on the product as to its suitability for you and your skin.

EYE MAKE-UP REMOVERS

If you wear eye make-up, you *must* use products specially designed for removing it. This is a thin-skinned, very delicate and sensitive area that we tend to lash with heavily pigmented, hard to remove make-up. Ordinary cleansers are not efficient at removing eye make-up and they can't cope with waterproof ones.

Clarins, who specialise in skin care products, discovered when testing eye care treatments that general cleansing and treatment products are too oily and can cause the mucous membrane under the eye to swell. So do use products specially formulated for this area and cleanse it first before working on the rest of your face. Use separate pads for each eye to avoid the risk of transmitting infection. Cleanse by moving from browbone down over lids to lashes in one sweep. The product removes the make-up – never rub or treat this area roughly.

EXFOLIATORS

Exfoliating products and facial scrubs are intended to even out the natural and continuous shedding of dead cells on the surface of the skin. After use, skin looks lighter, brighter and feels smoother, and is more ready to benefit from other treatments or to take make-up well. There is certainly a place for them in many skin routines but don't get carried away by their success and go for overkill. Once a week is enough for most people. They are not always necessary for young skins which have a naturally efficient exfoliating process going for them. They should not be used on very delicate, easily irritated or disturbed (spotty) skins and oily skins can be over-stimulated by the use of exfoliators.

There are many different types of exfoliators, so choose according to your budget, fancy and skin. Most exfoliating creams contain either natural particles with a rough texture – such as ground fruit stones – or smoother, rounded synthetic granules (which are gentler for more delicate skins). Both are massaged over the skin and rinsed away with water. There is also a gentle peeling cream which is spread on the skin, left to dry, and rubbed away. Liquid exfoliants, sometimes called clarifiers, work chemically rather than mechanically and do a smooth, efficient job, but can be a little tough for many skins.

There are also many exfoliating pads, sponges and loofah discs or slices designed to be used with a cleanser of your choice. Some contain their own built-in cleanser, so you use them once and discard them. From a hygiene and skin care point of view, disposable ones are preferable. Complexion brushes or a clean, dry face flannel have a mild sloughing effect and can be used to smooth the skin gently. These should always be spotlessly clean.

FACE MASKS

Face masks or packs are another means of giving a little cleansing boost to your complexion and these days few of them will set into Kabuki-like masks that mean you need total privacy to avoid someone making you laugh and your mask crack up. By temporarily coating the skin's surface, masks increase local circulation – helping you to look pinker and fitter – and encourage sweating, so deeper impurities are brought on to the surface of skin. Some have additional benefits, such as moisturising, soothing, softening and oil absorption, but all have a good cleansing and revitalising effect. Choose one suited to your skin type and use according to instructions.

STEAMING

This is an effective, inexpensive way of giving your skin and your face an occasional, more thorough cleanse. It will encourage sweating which brings impurities to the skin's surface and increases superficial circulation, making skin look brighter and feel softer. Steaming will also make the skin

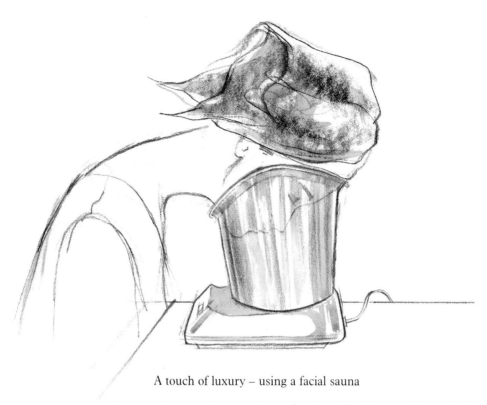

A touch of luxury – using a facial sauna

more receptive to other products, and professional facials usually include steaming before a face mask is applied.

Steaming is not advisable for sensitive skins with a tendency to redness or surface veins, and make-up should not be applied on any skin type for an hour or so after steaming. Best of all, have your treatment before you go to bed – it will prepare your skin beautifully for moisturiser. Here's how:

- Cleanse your face in the normal way, then add a litre or so of freshly boiled water to a bowl. Add a handful of fresh or dried herbs. Try rosemary, camomile or lavender, or buy a ready-made facial sauna pack and use according to the instructions.

- Hold your head about a foot away from the water. Drape a towel over your head and the basin to enclose the steam and stay like this for five to ten minutes.

- At the end of this time, rinse your face with warm water, blot dry with a clean towel, and apply a mask or moisturiser.

- Normal to oily skins can take this treatment twice a week, and normal to dry skins once a week.

MOISTURISING IS A MUST

Would you buy an expensive piece of furniture, stand it in a sunny window or by a radiator, knock it around a bit, never give it a touch of lubricating polish . . . and still expect it to look good in forty or fifty years time? Hardly, yet we can give this type of treatment to our faces – and far worse – on a daily basis.

Of course, we're not inanimate objects. What goes on inside our bodies, our general health, how our minds work, genetic tendencies, how we live and what our skin comes up against in life play a major role in the way it looks and whether it lasts well or lets us down with a bump at a fairly early age or several stages in our lives. But moisturisers can fulfil the polish role giving extra protection and helping the skin to look lustrous and well-cared for.

Moisture plays a large part in a youthful skin – a child's skin can have twice the water content of a very mature one – and balance is the factor that keeps it naturally moisturised. Water is constantly moving up from the lower layers of the epidermis to the *stratum corneum* (the outer layers of the skin) which contains a material known in the 'skin trade' as the natural moisturising factor (NMF). Water from the skin's surface is constantly evaporating into the atmosphere, but if the system is working well the natural moisturising factor helps to hold sufficient water in the outer layers to keep it smooth, supple and hydrated.

On the skin's surface sebum sweat and evaporating water from cells which have finished their lifespan mingle to form a natural emulsion called the hydro-lipidic film which is slightly acidic and protects the skin from attack by bacteria and pollution.

The wicked world and your own body are constantly attacking that beautiful natural skin balance. External hazards (wild weather, pollution, central heating, air conditioning, dabbling with harsh chemicals) and adverse internal conditions (from dodgy digestion, drastic dieting, illness, hormonal imbalances, negative stress, chemicals in food and medicines) can affect natural moisturising and sebum secretions. Sebum production, from the hormone-controlled sebaceous glands, starts to slow down at twenty or so (which can be a good thing if you're over-blessed with sebum production). For women, it falls quite considerably around thirty and does a dramatic drop after the menopause. Men always have a higher output which only declines slowly and steadily and the big drop-off doesn't happen until old age.

THE ROLE OF MOISTURISERS

Basically moisturisers are a back-up system for the body's own moisturising system and they help to keep the skin in an elegant condition when it's not working perfectly for itself. They sit on the skin's surface and help to prevent water from the surface evaporating too fast and improve the condition of the protective barrier. By smoothing down the outermost layers of cells (rather like hair conditioners smooth down roughed up 'tiles' on the outer layers of hair), they allow the skin to reflect light and look younger. Moisturised skin is slightly plumped up, so fine, dry lines are minimised. While a protected surface on the skin means it's better able to protect the lower layers, moisturisers do not nourish or feed your skin and they can't actually reverse what are generally known as age lines (although dermatologists may blame most of them on sun damage rather than the length of time you've been around).

When to start using moisturiser

When you begin to use a moisturiser has to be your own decision because only you know the state of your skin. Twenty-five should be a good starting point for most people, but many skins need to have help earlier than this. If there's the slightest hint of dryness, even if you're well under twenty-five, start immediately. As you grow older, and your skin becomes drier, it may need a richer product – again you'll have to be in charge of this decision.

How much you pay for your moisturiser is up to you, your financial state and what you feel is good for your skin (the power of the mind can't ever be divorced from body reaction). A world renowned American dermatologist praises the hydrating qualities of Vaseline. It may be efficient, and inexpensive, but could you stand that amount of grease on your face?

THE BASIC CHOICE

Water-in-oil

These creams are an upmarket version of Vaseline. They contain more oil than water and therefore do their job more efficiently and for far longer than oil-in-water moisturisers. They are formulated so they don't feel heavy and sticky on the skin, but nevertheless, their higher oil content makes them more suitable for night wear or dry or older skins. If you're inclined to dryness, it's also a good idea to wear them in cold, windy conditions outdoors or centrally heated (and therefore very dry) indoor atmospheres.

Oil-in-water

These moisturisers are light, easily absorbed products with a high water and low fat content. They make your skin feel good when you apply them, but the low oil content means the water soon evaporates and the length of their working time is limited. They're fine for young and/or oily skins and for day wear under make-up.

Oil-free

These moisturisers are based on a gel format that leaves the skin feeling soft and supple without adding extra grease, so they're a good choice for skins that have a tendency to oiliness, but from age or environmental conditions need moisturising and protecting.

Moisturisers containing UV filters

These are available in tinted or untinted versions and they're good walk-about day wear. You will probably need a sunscreen with a higher protection factor if you're out for any length of time in the hot sun. UV filters mean extra chemical ingredients, so don't wear them when it's not necessary. Give your face a rest from them in the evening or overnight by using a moisturiser containing no sunscreen ingredients.

MAKING THE MOST OF YOUR MOISTURISER

Apply moisturiser morning and night on a freshly-cleansed face and do add some during the day if you're in skin drying conditions. Massage it onto your face with light *upward* strokes, rather than just putting it on in a hit and miss fashion. Always use a rich water-in-oil emulsion at night if your skin is dry or mature and use throat cream or a rich water-in-oil emulsion on your neck before bed whatever your skin type. This can be a dry area even if the rest of your skin is quite oily.

Sensitive skins should have products containing no perfume or a hypo-allergenic product that is screened to be free from known irritants. If you're inclined to allergies, it's a good idea to choose products which list ingredients so anything that causes you trouble can soon be unmasked.

If you're acne prone – even if it hasn't been active for years – go for moisturisers (and cosmetics) which are described or advertised as non-comedogenic. In other words, those which are specifically formulated to avoid any substances likely to encourage blackheads and acne. Such formulations are a big thing in the States and, happily, are on the increase in Britain. Seek them out and keep break-outs at bay.

Blackheads and skin eruptions don't just happen overnight – they can take months to form – so the culprit could be a product you used some time ago, not your latest one.

Delicate zones

The eye area should be treated to its own special product. The skin around the eyes is particularly vulnerable, fragile, ultra-mobile, low in sebum and with a slightly different acid/alkali or pH balance from the rest of the skin. It can only tolerate low oil formulations or the mucous membrane under the eye swells like a damp sponge. So, eye treatment products should be low in oil content, perfume-free and non-irritant, and this is particularly important if you wear contact lenses or have sensitive eyes. Apply with great care using the third finger of your non-dominant hand (left if you're right handed, right if you're left handed) which ensures the lightest touch. Wash before touching the other eye to avoid any possibility of passing on infections.

Lips have no sebaceous glands, consequently they need plenty of rich water-in-oil moisturising or lip treatment cream/lip salve/lip protector, particularly in weather extremes.

Skin care and consideration hold back the lines of time, but whatever you do they arrive eventually. You can give your mouth a lift and ensure you have upward, outward moving lines around the eyes by looking on the brighter side of life as often as possible. Discontent and pessimism encourage a frown, a network of down-drooping lines around eyes and a tight 'miserable' mouth that's surrounded by tiny, vertical lines.

MORE FOR YOUR MOISTURE BALANCE

Moisturiser adds a degree of protection to your skin and helps when nature gives up a little on her task, but there are other ways to keep your own moisture balance at its best. It's wise to be wary of sun exposure (much more on this in chapter 5) and to follow a reasonably sensible lifestyle. Then try the following skin-kindly moves:

Keep up the humidity in your living and working conditions. Combat central heating, air conditioning and strip lighting with a humidifier or at least bowls of water around the room. Keep warm with a high tog duvet in winter, and turn down the heat in your bedroom.

Negative ions – the ones which abound on mountains and near moving water, such as the sea, rivers and streams – are known to have a calming effect, and have been used successfully to relieve a variety of ailments including migraines, and respiratory and skin problems. While the air we breathe is full of electrically charged particles called positive and negative

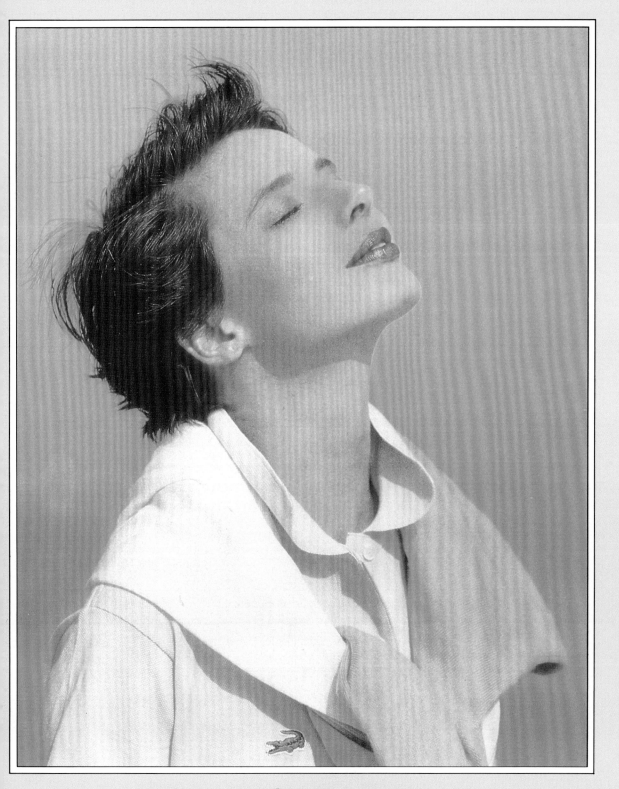

Beautiful skin.

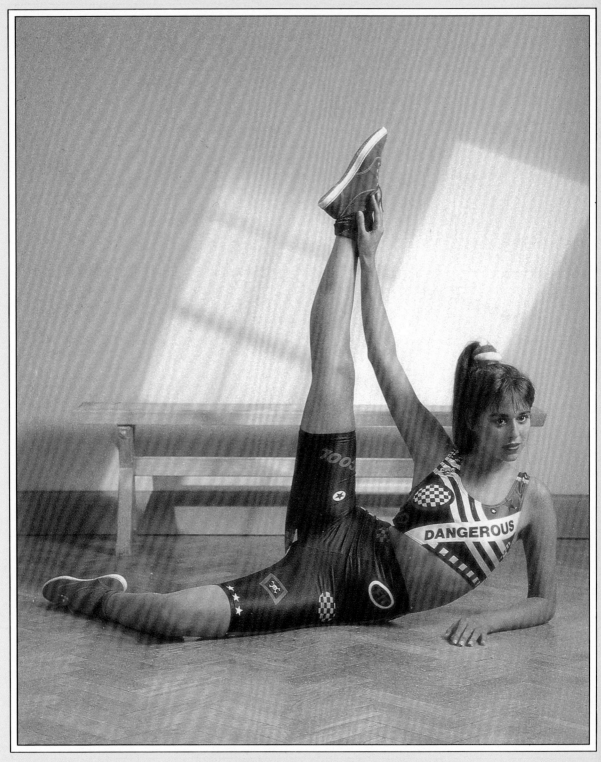

Exercise increases energy and the circulation and encourages relaxation
essential ingredients for a good skin.

ions, the proportion of positive ions increases when central heating, air conditioning and pollution are around. Ionisers, which help restore the balance, can be purchased to cover various sizes of room and can even be used in the car. The Japanese, who don't go in for half measures, used them in their workplaces and found that whilst people were feeling wonderful at work, they would fall into a deep depression as soon as they hit the polluted streets of Tokyo. Perhaps it's best not to over-cosset yourself, lest you can't cope with conditions outside, but an ioniser in the bedroom is certainly a good idea. It will help you to sleep more soundly, and breathe properly and it could be good for your skin.

Do keep up the internal water content. Drink several glasses of water each day – if you drink one before you go to sleep at night and one as soon as you wake in the morning, it can do a power of good for your body and your skin.

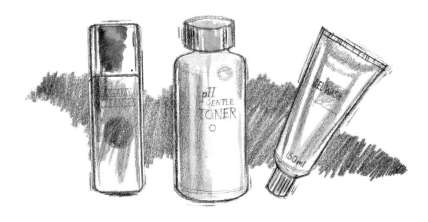

'MIRACLE' INGREDIENTS?

Years ago I spoke to a well-known dermatologist about 'miracle' ingredients then currently in skin care products. 'Secret substances collected from caves in Italy', he queried, 'What are they . . . bat's droppings?' 'Collagen!' he yelled, 'You might as well slap a piece of steak on your face.'

Well, science in skin care has moved apace since those days in search of products that will keep our skins looking as young as possible for as long as possible.

Basically, whether you pay out a pound or two or a tidy sum, a moisturiser sits on the surface of your skin and works by adding protection and helping to prevent evaporation of the skin's natural moisture content. When cosmetic doses of drugs are added to the moisturising formula – often described as active ingredients – the potential for penetration of the upper layers of the skin is higher.

Certainly, the larger, smarter and richer French and American cosmetic companies are walking innovative paths in formulating their anti-ageing products. So, if you've been bewildered by the science of beauty in the last few years, let's take a look at some of the ingredients now found in the more expensive products – and their possible action against the ageing process.

Liposomes

Liposomes are minute fluid-filled spheres made of the same phospholipids that constitute cell membranes. Their infinitely small size allows them to penetrate in between the cells of the *stratum corneum* to the skin's living cells where they act as delivery parcels releasing their active elements wherever and whenever they're needed and helping to 'Promote cell renewal, protect the cellular membrane and reform intercellular cement. In other words, they promise to hold back the ageing process.

Hyaluronic acid

This is a powerful, natural moisturiser with a structure that's suited to the liposome environment. Used medically to protect and lubricate – for instance in certain eye operations and to lubricate arthritic joints – it's now an active ingredient in some anti-ageing products.

Anti-oxidants and free radicals

You may have heard a great deal about 'free radicals'. Basically, they are the 'good guys' who turn bad. They are needed for such metabolic functions as oxygen absorption, energy production and the smooth working of the immune system. But once their job is finished, they're cast off by the molecules they were once part of and roam around looking for a resting place. They're prime enemies of the immune system and are thought to play a vicious role in premature ageing of the skin. Anti-oxidants (often forms of vitamins A, C or E or some of the trace minerals) provide a home for free radicals instead of letting these little age-makers run riot. Anti-oxidants are found in many of the latest sunscreens and skin care products. When used in very low concentrations, their function is to preserve the product and they are unlikely to do anything for your skin.

Retinoic acid

Retinoic acid or Retin-A is a derivative of vitamin A that has been used for years in the treatment of acne where it thins the epidermis, opens up follicles so oil can drain to the surface and speeds up cell turnover. It has been found that in some cases it made skin look younger and reversed some of the results of sun damage like uneven pigmentation and the thickening of the skin's surface layers that gives that leathery, weather-beaten look. A cosmetic version of the active ingredient of retinoic acid, called vitamin A Palmitate, is being used successfully by some companies in liposome-delivering, anti-ageing products.

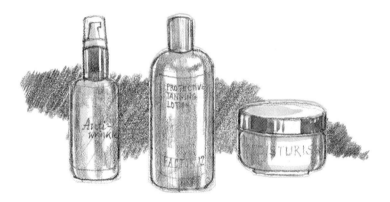

NATURAL INGREDIENTS

Ingredients don't have to be world-shatteringly new to act as first class moisturisers and some houses are leaning heavily towards moisturising ingredients that have been used to soothe and smooth skin for centuries:

Jojoba

Jojoba is a liquid wax obtained from the seeds of a shrub native to Mexico and some southern US states. Jojoba is able to flourish in some of the poorest land in the world. It has been used for centuries by American Indians for skin and scalp disorders. It is the only plant yet known which produces a natural liquid wax almost identical in composition to sperm whale oil previously used in moisturising products, so environmentally involved people like the Body Shop are delighted to use it in products to help save that endangered species.

Aloe Vera

Aloe Vera grows wild in the tropics and is now cultivated in many sub-tropical climates. Its cactus-like leaves (in fact it's a member of the lily family) are filled with yellow juice which contains the bitter-tasting aloes drug. It has been used for thousands of years in medicinal and cosmetic preparations – Cleopatra was reputed to keep her complexion clear and soft with it, and it was certainly used to treat radiation burns at Hiroshima and Nagasaki. When sufficient amounts are used in skin care formulations, it stimulates circulation and soothes, protects and moisturises skin.

Oil of evening primrose

Oil of Evening Primrose helps the skin to retain moisture. For more information on this plant see page 77.

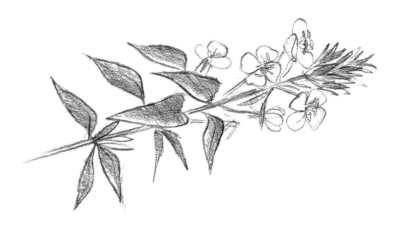

Cocoa butter

Cocoa butter comes from the roasted, pressed seeds of the cacao tree which grows in tropical climates. South Sea Islanders use it to moisturise their skin and scalp and the actress Mae West reputedly covered herself from top to toe with it every night. It's an excellent skin softener and moisturiser.

COMING TO TERMS

When you see a label making play of the kind-to-skin properties of a beauty product, do you always know what it means? The following tips might help.

Allergy Screened   Each ingredient in the product has passed through stringent tests to ensure that it has the minimum possible history of causing any allergic reactions.

Dermatologically Tested   The product has been patch tested on the skin of a panel of human volunteers (who are usually chosen for their sensitive skins) to monitor it for any tendency to cause irritation.

Hypo-allergenic   These products are usually fragrance and alcohol free, contain the minimum colouring agents and no known irritants or sensitisers. That is not a total guarantee that no-one will have an allergic reaction to them. Someone, somewhere can be allergic to anything – even water.

Lanolin Free   Lanolin is an excellent skin moisturiser and softener and as it is obtained from sheep's wool it is relatively inexpensive. Unfortunately, it is a well-known allergen and can encourage blackheads, whiteheads etc. Some beauty houses now make much of the absence of lanolin in their products.

Non-comedogenic   This is a current buzz-term, particularly for products aimed at the younger end of the market. It means that the product has been screened to eliminate ingredients that will clog the follicles and encourage blackheads and whiteheads (open and closed comedones).

pH Balanced   This is accepted as the norm these days in most cosmetic and toiletry products. The pH scale measures the acidity or alkalinity of a solution with 7 as neutral; any number below that showing increasing acidity. Numbers above 7 show increasing alkalinity with 14 as the top strength. Healthy skin has a slightly acidic reading, so pH balanced products are slightly acidic to maintain the natural healthy mantle of fatty acid. Alkaline products tend to strip this acid mantle and leave the skin vulnerable for a certain amount of time.

YOUR GUIDE TO A SKIN CARE ROUTINE

The operative word here is 'guide'. Skin behaviour and reaction is very individual and a routine that's perfect for one person with a certain type of skin may not work so well for another with the same skin type. Try the suggested routine for your skin category on the next two pages, but feel free to change anything that doesn't seem to be working well for you.

YOUR GUIDE TO A SKIN CARE ROUTINE

DAILY ROUTINE	Normal Skin	Dry Skin
CLEANSING morning	cleansing milk/ cleansing bar/rinse off cleanser/lotion	cleansing milk/lotion
evening (if you wear foundation)	gel/lotion/cream cleanser	lotion/cream cleanser
Eye make-up remover	√	√
TONING	√	√
MOISTURISING morning	tinted or oil-in-water moisturiser	tinted or water-in-oil moisturiser
evening	oil-in-water moisturiser	water-in-oil moisturiser
Eye balm/gel moisturiser	√	√
Lip moisturiser/ treatment cream	√	√
Body moisturiser	√	√

EXTRAS

	Normal Skin	Dry Skin
EXFOLIATING (face & body) Gentle scrub	1 a week	2 a month
FACE MASK Toning	1 a week	×
Moisturising mask	○	2 a week
SUNSCREENING (wherever and whenever necessary)	√	√

KEY TO SYMBOLS	√ use	× don't use	○ use if necessary

Dry/Sensitive Skin	Oily Skin	Combination Skin
Cleansing milk/lotion/ cream cleanser	cleansing bar/rinse-off cleanser	cleansing bar/rinse-off cleanser
gel/lotion/cream cleanser	rinse-off lotion/gel	rinse-off lotion
√	√	√
√	√	√
tinted or water-in-oil moisturiser	oil-free moisturiser	tinted or oil-free moisturiser
water-in-oil moisturiser	oil-free moisturiser	oil-in-water moisturiser
√	√	√
√	√	√
√	avoid chest and back if very oily	√

×	1 a week (unless very oily/blemished)	1 a week
×	1 a week	1 a week
2 a week	×	○
√	√	√

WHEN TRYING NEW PRODUCTS

If you are buying and trying new skin care products or cosmetics, give them a chance! Don't use them for the first time:

- in the few days prior to a period. Wait until it's over and by the time the next one is around, your skin will have acclimatised to the new product – if it needs to.

- when you've been on any sort of medication, particularly some form of antibiotic which can temporarily throw your immune system out of balance.

- if you're having dental treatment that includes injections and x-rays, which can make your skin ultra-sensitive.

- when you've any form of respiratory trouble including a chesty cold.

- when you first go on holiday and your body is adjusting to many different conditions.

- when you've been ill, had an operation or during a particularly stressful time in your life.

Changing to a new type of skin care routine, for instance using a cleanser and toner when you've used soap and water before, may initially bring out a spot or two because your skin is being stimulated (which is good). Generally, you will find that it will adjust to the new regime very quickly. If any adverse skin reaction lasts for more than a few days when you're using a new product, return to the consultant for advice. You may be using it wrongly or too vigorously.

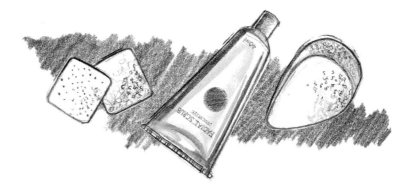

Skin care for a lifetime

Very young skin

After months of lumbering around heavily pregnant, a mother gives birth. Even the least sentimental of us will admit that the whole process is a major miracle. Out the baby pops – or struggles – often looking somewhat worse for the journey and along with the thrill and the sense of achievement, there's anxiety, particularly if it's the first major production.

How will we cope with this small person who depends on us for its existence? And often, even doting new parents will query those looks. 'Where's that soft, beautiful skin we hear so much about?' they say . . . 'My baby looks like a wrinkled little old person covered in blotches, strange marks and – heavens – hair in the wrong places!'

If you've any worries about your baby, including its skin, your doctor, midwife, nurse, health visitor or clinic will give you all the answers and help you need, but it's as well to have some idea of what you might expect.

Before a baby is born, it's cosseted in a dark, warm and enclosed place, kept at a constant temperature, and protected from most dangerous substances. Suddenly, he or she is thrust into the world . . . and skin plays a big part in keeping a young baby safe in this very strange, new environment. As with adult's skin it prevents harmful substances from getting to the body and its temperature control function is vital to this very new body.

At birth, a baby is usually covered with vernix, a substance rather like cream cheese in appearance, which has protected the skin before birth and continues doing so for a few hours after birth until it's absorbed or the excess is wiped away. The amount of downy hair (*laguna*) on a newborn baby – particularly some premature ones – can sometimes be a shock. Again, this is a leftover from development in the womb, and will disappear within a matter of days.

The bluish skin when a baby appears soon changes to a healthy pink shade as its own circulatory system gets going, but the extremities – hands and feet – may take longer. Jaundice affects something like fifty per cent of babies, so your newborn child might be distinctly yellowish a couple of days after birth.

Mothers who feel that birth was a big effort might give a thought to the struggle a tiny baby has to put up during the process. Blotches, scratches, bruises, pressure marks and puffy eyelids are sometimes a leftover from time in the womb and the fight to get out into the world. Enlarged oil glands and acne-like spots are not uncommon and are probably a legacy of the mother's hormonal activity. Most skin imperfections clear up on their own accord within a matter of weeks after birth.

Distinct blue veins may be visible on the body, temples and bridge of nose, particularly on fine-skinned babies, and they may remain obvious for several months. Darker skinned babies of Mediterranean, Asian or Afro-Caribbean descent may have bruise-like marks on their lower back (Mongolian Blue Spots) until they are past toddler stage.

Many tiny babies have a greasy look on the skin around their eyes and this can last until the tear ducts start working when they're a few weeks old. (This shouldn't be confused with a sticky eye infection which is a discharge from the eye and is a minor, common infection that needs medical attention.)

Some babies start life with a beautiful skin and then it may peel a little. They may develop a few yellowish spots on the face where immature oil glands have not completely opened. Little rashes may develop due to heat (high summer temperatures or too much clothing in winter) or irritation when that very delicate skin rubs on clothing and sheets. Use gentle soap flakes rather than detergents to wash baby and bed clothes and choose natural rather than synthetic fibres and good baby products formulated to maintain normal healthy skin flora. Non-perfumed, allergy tested, pH balanced oils, lotions or creams are important assets in looking after this delicate skin.

Cradle cap, which looks a bit like dandruff, may appear on the soft top of a baby's head when it's a few weeks old. A little baby oil and shampoo should keep this under control, and again, it will disappear of its own accord at three to four months of age.

Nappy rash is an occupational hazard in babies due to their evacuation habits and the hothouse atmosphere produced by plastic pants and leak-proof nappies. Make sure you allow plenty of bare bottom kicking time, do plenty of nappy changing and use a good baby cream.

Coping with a new baby for the first time is rather like learning anything new – you've been shown how to do things, but you'll still feel nervous and will inevitably make mistakes. Aim to get the most enjoyment out of it even if it means cutting corners in the early days – doing things like just washing essential places if bathtime makes you both fraught. And if you can't think where all the time goes, forget the finer points of housework for a month or so. Don't work yourself to a frazzle trying to keep things as they were – it's not worth it.

New babies are fragile, but they're not meant to be wrapped in cotton wool. A healthy baby needs fresh air and should go out every day (except in fog), suitably clothed and protected from insects, animals, cold, heat, rain, wind and, most important, the sun.

Apart from the fact that young skins haven't spent time 'toughening up' to cope with the elements, their skin is different in composition to that of adults and young people. Pound for pound, the skin level of very young babies has a higher water content, different mineral levels, and far less collagen. These all more or less even up by six to seven months, but sebum levels in babies and small children are much lower than in adults – production increases fourfold between the ages of six and fifteen.

The dangers of sunning are emphasised in chapter 5. Babies and young children are particularly susceptible to the sun and their cells are developing and dividing and are very easily damaged. Do protect them at all times.

Most new parents learn to relax and natural pride and enjoyment outweigh anxiety when a baby reaches three to four months old and is more a little person, less like a delicate, floppy doll. While it may seem a massive jump from infancy to puberty, life is usually not too complicated on the skin front until the dreaded puberty strikes. Your child becomes an adolescent with all the physical (and don't let's think about emotional) changes involved in this complicated process. One of the more obvious features is that your child's fresh, enviable complexion is very likely to become greasy, and coarser (particularly in males), and prone to blackheads and eruptions to a more or less distressing degree.

Don't scream at this point if you're in your twenties, thirties, forties and even fifties and still coping with major outbreaks of spots. Acne can be a fight all your life or it can crop up for the first time later in life. But it's usually thought of as a teenage trouble along with all the other problems that puberty brings.

TEENAGE TROUBLES

Acne – or some degree of blemished skin – usually explodes into our lives at a time of maximum emotional insecurity. Sex hormones rise and suddenly loud and confident little girls and boys become even louder, self-conscious semi-adults with uncoordinated limbs, mercurial emotions and – according to their sex – the traumas of first periods and new-found curves or embryonic beards on baby faces and voices that boom and squeak in one short sentence.

The transition from child to grown-up rarely rolls smoothly and to crown it all, there are – in something like seventy per cent of pubescent people – surges of obvious oil, spots and sometimes wicked, red, painful lumps and pustules on face and upper body. In most cases (certainly not all) the condition peaks in the late teens and dies a natural death in the early twenties, but it can leave behind a legacy of scarred skin and crumpled confidence. In the meantime, big steps such as getting a job, going on to higher education, growing awareness of the opposite sex, and general social interaction as an adult have to be coped with while facing the world with a blemished skin, and the low self-image and stress that can bring.

Why do some people manage to avoid any obvious greasy-faced stage, some have oily skin and no blemishes, others suffer anything from a minor to a major breakdown in their skin's smooth functioning? While all the answers aren't yet known, it appears that acne is yet another genetic problem – in other words, it tends to run in families.

Other spot producing factors involved are the hormones testosterone and progesterone, which provide fuel for acne-prone skin. Testosterone is the hormone responsible for stimulating the development of the sebaceous follicles and getting the oil flowing. But while the acne-prone may wish it didn't exist, it plays a vital part in sexual development. It's the major male sex hormone which, in men, promotes bone and muscle growth, deep voices and beards. Female ovaries, along with oestrogen and progesterone, produce small amounts of testosterone. In both men and women it's a vital ingredient in their sexual drive.

While the oil may flow with little more trouble than inconvenience and a shiny face, in the acne-inclined, there may be an increase in cell renewal, and in any case, as acned skin is sticky, shedding of the lining cells of the follicle doesn't happen in the normal way. Trapped in their little pits, sticky dead cells and more oil get together in a solid mass plugging the follicle. Bacteria thrive in these conditions, and that's when trouble can start.

Whiteheads or closed comedones, are plugs of hardened sebum, dead cells and debris with skin cells closing off the follicle exit, so you get what looks like a white spot under the skin's surface Flex your lower lip, and if your skin is oily, you're likely to see some minor examples in the horizontal cleft of your chin.

Blackheads have the same composition, but the follicle exit is open. The black appearance is not caused by dirt, but by oil that has oxidised on contact with air plus some pigment granules.

Acne comes in many degrees, from skins with some whiteheads, some blackheads and the occasional inflamed spot on a face to cases where face, back, chest and shoulders can be a mass of blackheads, whiteheads, inflamed pustules and angry red lumps.

When a spot becomes inflamed, it will often die down of its own accord in a matter of days if left strictly alone. But certain conditions, such as being tired, stressed, feeling off-colour, fiddling with the spot or sometimes just being the unproud owner of an erupting skin with all the misery and stress this brings, can make a pustule out of a pimple or start a new eruption. White blood cells rush in to fight the inflammation and pus forms near the surface of the skin. Sometimes the whole swollen, inflamed mass may cause the follicle wall to blow out and the debris can be dumped into the dermis, leaving a deep seated lump with no outlet – one that can flare up again at any time. When the follicle wall ruptures there is usually some scarring.

ACNE CONTROL

There is, as yet, no cure for acne, but it can be controlled by various means, and it's vital to inhibit the development of inflamed spots that can lead to scarring and permanent reminders of the problem. If you are a teenager or many years older with a susceptibility to skin eruptions work along these lines:

- **Be scrupulously clean,** but don't keep dabbing at your face. Two thorough cleanses a day – morning and evening – are fine. Wash and rinse your hands before you touch your face and rinse off every trace of cleansing product with plenty of clean, warm water. Shampoo hair frequently and keep it well away from your face.

- **Keep additional oil to a minimum.** Avoid any oil in hairdressings. If you need or want to use moisturiser, go for one that is labelled non-comedogenic or use a skin gel rather than a cream or lotion. Choose an oil-free, water-based foundation and loose powder – pressed powder can contain oil. Remove make-up when you are spending time at home alone – unless it makes you feel depressed to see your skin uncovered!

- **Treat blackheads** and whiteheads with an exfoliating scrub a couple of times a week using a clean, dry flannel, a complexion brush, exfoliating puff, or gentle scrubbing grains unless your face has inflamed blemishes or is very oily when it can be too harsh and stimulating.

- **Steam clean** and use a toning mask on your face once a week unless you are having medical treatment for your blemishes. In that case, ask your doctor if it's a wise move for you or not.

- **Hands off!** Unprofessional picking, squeezing and prodding at blemishes will only make them worse. You risk spreading bacteria and leaving behind some of the debris so the area will flare up again, or forcibly bursting the follicle wall and possibly causing real problems.

- **Stop habit handling** – such as rubbing your chin, or leaning your cheek on one hand.

- **Eat well,** and eat early. While good dietary habits don't prevent or cure acne, bad ones can increase your stress potential and irritate the problem. Try to have a good breakfast, a good lunch and finish eating for the day by six pm if possible. Never eat snacks in the late evening or just before bed. If you suspect an allergy to any foods, try to avoid them. Eating the occasional hamburger may do little harm from the inside but letting the grease run down onto your chin may be adding fuel to the chin spot syndrome.

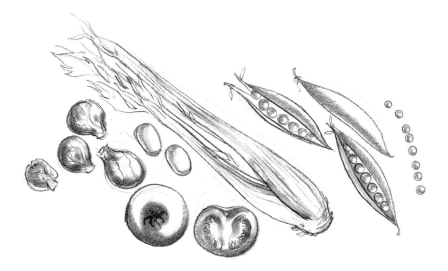

- **Try a zinc supplement** – up to 100 mg a day. It will certainly do you no harm and where there is inflammation, it seems to reduce it in some cases.

- **Cut out artificial stimulants** if you seriously want to get to grips with skin blemishes – cigarettes, coffee, caffeinated drinks. Keep alcohol consumption low too.

- **Avoid prolonged stress** as much as possible – it stimulates hormone production. Get plenty of exercise, sleep, relaxation, fresh food, fresh air and fun.

- **Enjoy your holidays.** Gentle sunshine, fresh air, exercise and fun help people to relax – which may bring a double bonus for acne sufferers and improve their skins. A *gentle* tan will camouflage superficial scars as well. However, you may be unlucky. Dermatologists reckon about twenty-five per cent of acne cases are made worse by sunlight – and that percentage increases in humid conditions.

- **Over the pharmacist's counter** preparations abound, but there is a treatment gel on the market which contains *Ethyl Lactate* (with zinc sulphate). This reduces bacteria and inflammation without being tough on the skin or drying it out excessively. Testers found it did a good job on mild, localised acne.

- **Find a sympathetic doctor/dermatologist** if your spots are more than very occasional little outbursts. Current treatment may include one or more of the following:

The oestrogen content in certain birth control pills helps to control sebum output and can be a help to female sufferers. It's no go for men, who would develop breasts, voice and beard changes along with any improvement in their acne.

Benzoyl peroxide in water based gels acts by peeling surface skin, prevents blocked follicles, suppresses irritating fatty acids in sebum, and fights bacteria.

Retinoic acid (vitamin A acid) is a great peeler, and can be useful in some cases where there are many closed comedones.

Low dose antibiotics taken orally over a period of time are often successful at suppressing acne. Externally applied antibiotics may be prescribed.

13-cis-retinoic acid (trade name in the UK – Roaccutane) a related, but slightly different chemical compound to retinoic acid has a high success rate. But, as it's extremely expensive and has quite severe side effects at times (including the possibility of birth defects if a woman becomes pregnant while taking it) its use is limited to very severe acne cases.

Isolutrol, the most recent discovery which may help in the battle against over-active sebaceous glands and acne, has what sounds like a bizarre origin – sharks' bile. It is thought that the bile acids which emulsify fats in sharks' bodies are the basis of its success. The ingredient has now been synthetically replicated and controlled volunteer studies have shown that it greatly reduces oiliness. It is marketed in Britain as Solution 28 and is being used in clinical trials.

Adult acne

In rare cases acne continues through to middle age or beyond, but some people develop acne for the first time in their twenties, thirties or forties. This often follows a severe shock, or a period of intense stress and strain. Pregnant women can sometimes develop acne in the early months, but this usually subsides in the later months.

Pre-period outbreaks are very common and probably due to high pro-gesterone levels at that time. If you have a tendency to retain water, come out in spots or generally feel bloated and unattractive during the run up to menstruation, try dipping into potassium rich foods for at least a week before – bananas, tomatoes, avocados, or fresh or dried apricots. At the very least, this regime tends to curb any craving for the 'quick lift' that comes from sugary snacks and chocolate.

Getting rid of after effects

If the skin is scarred, chemical peeling or dermabrasion may be used to minimise or remove scarring on burnt-out cases of acne. Pits and valleys can sometimes be filled in with liquid collagen. If at all possible, it is better to get medical advice and treatment early and this may help you to avoid scarring.

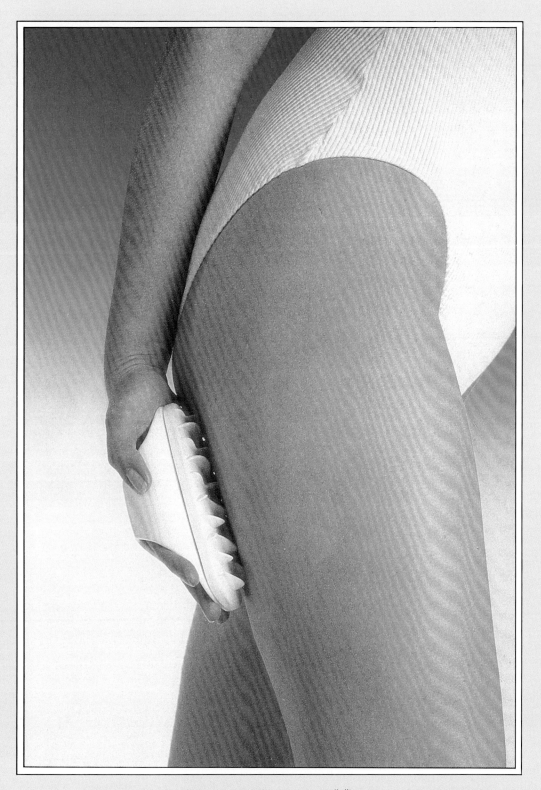

Massage can help to remove cellulite.

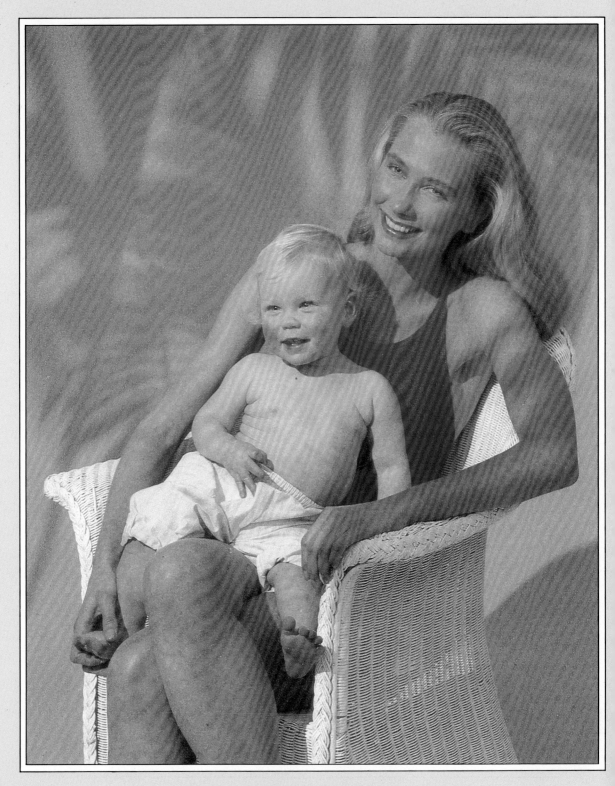

Babies and young children have delicate skins which must be carefully looked after.

GROWING OLDER

Have you been through the trauma yet? The shock when you see that first unflattering photograph that shows your wrinkles in fine relief, or a new-angle glimpse of your face that hints of falls to come, the realisation that your friends are looking a little ancient – can they be thinking the same about you?

Ageing does seem to happen overnight. But this is not the case. From about the mid-twenties onwards it's a very slow, progressive, and inevitable process.

If you're in your teens or twenties, don't skip this section. Although you can't imagine being a wrinkly, and ten or twenty years seems a lifetime away, most of this advice can't be taken too soon if you want to put your best face forward for life. Of course, good health, a sensible, reasonably fortunate life-style, internal and external skin care and genetic good luck do play an important role.

Spring from a family that ages well and you've chalked up bonus anti-ageing marks. Good, shapely cheekbones, a strong jawline, a fairly resilient, bouncy skin and your face is far less likely to collapse before its time. Delicate skin stretched tightly over the bony understructure can look wonderful in youth, but just about everything in the environment will steal its moisture content and lash it with lines all too soon in life. At the other extreme, a fleshy face with poor muscle tone and flattish bone structure will follow the rules of gravity and fall into jowls and pouches. Some faces have quite defined 'character' lines even in youth – from nose to mouth, on the forehead above a very mobile brow and at the sides of eyes, and these etch more deeply as the years go by.

Most illnesses, medical conditions and drugs affect the skin and make it less able to function well for you. For instance, diabetics have a tendency to skin infections and eruptions, and stress can encourage acne; under-active thyroid, rough, dry skin. Some antibiotics cause increased sensivity to ultraviolet light, and antihistamines and frequent doses of diuretics and laxatives will dehydrate the skin. Oriental diagnosis believes the lungs and skin to be sister organs – a theory not to be scoffed at with the high incidence of sensitive, dried out skins found in polluted places. Certainly, a cared for body that spends its life in the country is likely to bear the passing years more easily than an equally cared for one that's subject to the stress and pollution of large town living. Britain's relatively damp and temperate conditions are kinder to skins than dry and tropical or sub-tropical climates or parts of the world with extremes of heat and cold.

The ageing process of the face is the same as for the rest of the body, but it's a more delicate skin than that on your back and buttocks, yet it's out there exposed for every day of your life while tougher parts are covered and protected.

Imperceptibly and very slowly, the skin thins and the elastic fibres of the dermis become less resilient. As they fall into furrows around areas where there's muscle movement, the epidermis follows their fall, so you'll have more wrinkles around very mobile areas like the eyes and mouth than you will on cheeks. The metabolic processes slow down with age, so consequently sebum production drops and the inter-cellular cement of the skin is less efficient. Gradually, the skin dries out. Muscle tone is less effective and the skeletal frame shrinks a little.

Men's skins are naturally thicker, tougher and oilier than women's, so the ageing process is slower. But men tend to take less care care of their skins. (See pages 56–60 for specific advice.)

For both men and women external care – cleansing, moisturising, exfoliating, wearing clothes and products which will protect them from ultra violet rays – and internal care are vital to youthful looks, but there's even more positive good we can do for ourselves:

- **Avoid the diet see-saw.** Stay as closely as possible to your ideal weight. Months of moaning about how fat you're getting, and a mad crash diet to lose a stone three weeks before your holiday will leave skin like a punctured balloon. (Doesn't weight always fall away from your face first, and cling like mad to areas you want to slim?) Unbalanced nutrition leads to dried-up skin. If you're overweight, get rid of the excess slowly and sensibly, and keep your body toned with exercise.

- **A glass of wine** with an evening meal can be one of life's pleasures, helps you to relax with friends, savour your food better and eat more slowly. But regular, heavy drinking is poison. The warm glow a drink brings to your skin can, with time, turn into a mess of sluggish capillaries – a blotchy, red complexion will be the end result. Alcohol is a depressant, and heavy drinking increases stress. It reduces the body's absorption of vitamins and batters your liver which, among other horrors, leads to dried out, prematurely aged and pouchy skin. If you have a weight problem, remember each glass is full of empty calories – no real nutrients.

- **Constipation** can dull the complexion, and make you look and feel sluggish. Make sure elimination is thorough as well as regular. It's a very good idea to put your feet on a little footstool when you're sitting on the lavatory – the sort you can buy in some maternity shops – so you're in a more natural position to aid elimination.

- **Smoking** is a major health hazard. It does nothing for your skin either. It hampers your breathing capacity which in turn hampers circulation and leads to oxygen starvation of skin cells, an unlively texture and premature wrinkles. If you're still a smoker, light up your next one in front of a mirror and see what happens to your face as you view through a smoke haze – eyes and forehead crinkle up, the mouth puckers around the cigarette. You've seen what smoke does to a kipper – it's doing the same for your skin.

- **Your dentist is good for your looks.** Bad teeth and infected gums may lead to outbreaks of spots and losing your natural teeth is a prime ager as this will encourage the development of jowls, lines around the lips, and loss of lip shape. Work with your dentist to find the best ways to keep your mouth healthy. Have six-monthly checkups and any repair or reconstruction work your dentist suggests.

- **Your optician can keep you looking younger.** Check that you're not frowning and screwing up your eyes in order to see more clearly – short sighted people automatically narrow the amount of light coming through the pupils to increase the depth of focus. *Presbyopia* strikes around forty. The muscles of the eyes gradually become less efficient. Again, difficulty with focussing leads to facial contortions as you find the small print impossible to read if it's held less than an arm's length away. Get your eyesight checked regularly, and do wear your glasses and contact lenses if you need to.

- **Necks can raddle before faces** and many people spend half their lives bent over worktops and with the head and neck held badly as they walk and move. Hold the neck straight whenever possible. Pillows should support your head without raising it so far that you're curving your neck and doubling your chin.

- **Forget face workouts.** Unless you've taken a vow of silence or your face is incredibly immobile, it gets enough exercise without adding to its constant movement and wrinkling potential with a facial muscle workout. Indeed some exercises suggested for neck and chin firming over-strengthen the *platysma* muscle (the one that runs down the front of the neck), so it stands out like two cords down your throat, and can look very ugly.

- **Neck exercises.** The neck routine given opposite is the exception to the rule, as it relaxes the area, and wards off dowager's hump and upper spine problems. Do ten of each of these in the mornings, and try to fit in a few during the day if you have a sedentary job:

- **Big busts** should be kept in place with an expertly fitted bra. Without firm support, breasts can follow the laws of gravity, and may stretch the skin of your neck and jawline as they droop.

- **The menopause** must be mentioned in any discussion of age I suppose, but worrying about possible problems is often as bad as any real physical ones you may have. Your skin doesn't dry up and fall into furrows overnight at any time of your life, but if oestrogen levels drop suddenly this can affect sebaceous glands and moisture levels and feeling anxious and unwell will reflect in the face. Regular visits to a sympathetic gynaecologist are a must.

- **Stay in step** with physical and fashion changes in your looks. Skin and hair lighten as you grow older. You may not be putting the white hairs on show, but don't have them coloured to your original shade – go lighter or streaked to complement your lighter skin tones. It is important to keep up with make-up trends, don't stick to the same look for years – nothing is more ageing and dating. Make-up is looking increasingly natural today, and it's a look that's much more flattering to mature faces than lashings of cosmetics.

- **Enjoy a mini facelift** even if you don't have the money or inclination for cosmetic surgery. Try one of the beauty creams or ampoules that reduce lines, firm your face for a few hours and provide a smoother surface for make-up. They contain a high concentration of hydrating agents and collagen which sits on the skin's surface and fills in fine lines.

- **Be happy.** A smile makes you look friendly, approachable and full of life. It's catching, and will make everyone around you happier. Laughter is an exercise that moves muscles in your chest and diaphragm, increases your lung power and circulation and reduces stress. Anger, depression and discontent use muscles that drag down the face and mouth. Smiles and laughter use major lifting muscles from lip corner to cheekbones. So smiling and laughing will actually make you look younger, and feel better. Try it out for yourself.

Neck exercises

1. With chin parallel to the ground, look first left then right, moving your head slowly and trying to get the chin past your shoulder each time.

2. Slowly relax the head forward, then straighten up.

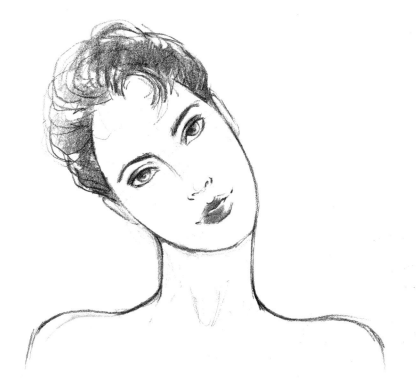

3. Look ahead with neck straight, try to touch the right shoulder with the right ear, then the left shoulder with the left ear.

4. Look straight ahead and push your head forward keeping shoulders still (it makes you look a bit like an emerging tortoise), then pull it back as far as possible.

- **Sinus problems** can hamper good breathing habits, and can lead to veins on cheeks and pouchy faces. Clear yours – before you raise your head from the pillow in the morning (see opposite).

AGEING – WAYS TO AVOID IT?

Let's not play with Retin-A

Retinoic acid (trade name Retin-A) is a drug that has been used in gels for years in the treatment of acne to stimulate circulation, speed cell turnover, thin the epidermis and open up closed comedones in order to allow the combination of dead cells, oil and junk to escape instead of filling the follicles to bursting point. Along the way it can cause reddened, irritated, thinner skin that should be treated with care, with gentle products and kept out of the sun.

It can also – after a period of treatment – inhibit production of uneven pigment, so skin tone may become more even and the skin looks lustier and younger. Currently, Retin-A is causing a touch of hysteria in many non-medical circles and is being acclaimed as the long-awaited product that will keep us all looking young for years longer.

But, retinoic acid is *not* magic. In fact, its action is quite fierce, and it can't be considered a foolproof panacea for ageing. With normal ageing – and this happens to everyone sooner or later according to their genetic make-up – the skin thins. When the skin is exposed overmuch to strong sunshine, we get photo-ageing where the skin thickens, bringing prematurely wrinkled, leathery looks.

Retin-A will not make old skin look young again. It could possibly have some beneficial effects for skin prematurely aged by sun damage. But it is hazardous to use it for more than a short period of time, or without clinical control, on fine, delicate and freckled skin – the very type that is likely to be prematurely aged by exposure to the sun. Everyone should be aware that this is a potent drug.

HRT – will it change your life?

During a woman's child-bearing years there is a delicate balance between the pituitary gland and the ovaries (which secrete oestrogen and progesterone) which results in the monthly reproductive cycle. Some time, usually between the ages of 40 and 55, the ovaries gradually cut down on oestrogen and progesterone production. Periods can become less frequent and sometimes heavy or light when they do happen. Eventually, they cease altogether which means that child-bearing days are over. Some bodies can

Sinus clearer

1. Place fingertips of both hands vertically on the centre of forehead, so little fingers are just above centre brow, forefingers just below hairline. Press, then slide fingers towards temples an inch, and press again. Repeat this press and slide with your fingers across the forehead, down the side of the temples, to the front of your ear, finishing just behind the ear.

2. With your forefinger just above your cheekbone, and thumb just below, start at the edge of your nose. Press, move out an inch, then press again. Repeat to the outer edge of the cheekbone, down the front of the ear and finish behind the earlobe.

3. Hold chin at centre point with thumbs behind, and fingers in front. Press and slide an inch. Repeat the move up the jawbone to the ear.

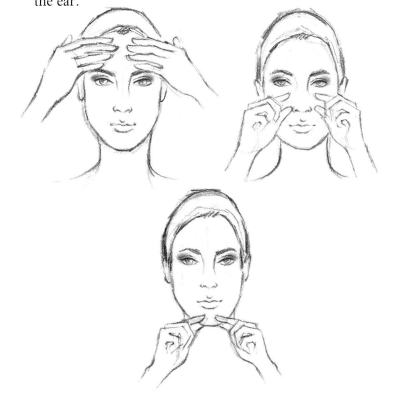

cope with this hormonal change, others don't do so well. Sometimes there can be side effects, which can include hot flushes, panic attacks, insomnia, lack of energy, depression, wild mood changes, loss of libido, skin problems (including adult acne) and loss of calcium from the bones which can lead to osteoporosis.

Uncomfortable and physically/mentally distressing symptoms can often be alleviated by Hormone Replacement Therapy (HRT). Oestrogen and progesterone (the progesterone reduces the risk of cancer of the lining of the uterus) may be taken orally in the form of a pill or introduced into the body via a cream, pessaries or an implant which releases a continuous supply. Women who have had a hysterectomy can have oestrogen alone. As they have no womb lining they don't need the progesterone. HRT can help many women over this hormonal hiccup in their lives. For others, it will do nothing at all or will even make them feel ill. It is certainly not a 'stay young forever' potion. It should not be taken if you have very few or no ill effects during the menopause (many women hardly notice it happening) and, although you will take HRT with your GP's or gynaecologist's advice, doctors do not know in advance how your body will react to it. Without doubt a sensible lifestyle, a contented mind and spirit, and plenty of interest in life are the best form of medicine to help you through this time.

MEN – A CHANGE OF FACE

Have you noticed the quiet revolution that's been going on in the past few years? Gone are the days when a self-respecting man would sooner smell of perspiration than perfume and the idea of using a moisturiser or having a beauty treatment would have got him laughed out of the pub or club. Henry Cooper 'splashed it all over' back in the seventies and the concept of pleasant-smelling men who cared about themselves took off.

Today, men have come out into the open, and no longer surreptitiously use the moisturiser belonging to the woman in their lives (if they do borrow, they're blatant about it) or blame their fragrance on gifts from the girls. While the young and fashionable males still provide the largest slice of buying power, it's boom time for sales of men's grooming aids, and skin cleansers and moisturisers for men have made an appearance in major chain stores – a sign that they're likely to be best sellers.

Fashion has something to do with it – the androgynous looks of the seventies have at least re-vamped the old woollen sweater and beer belly image, and health, fitness and grooming are now considered important. The present social scenario with high unemployment everywhere has squashed the myth that wrinkles in males are rugged – looking young and vital helps you to get or keep your job whatever your sex.

It is true that men start with a natural, stay-young advantage when it comes to skin. Among all the other changes that happen at puberty, their skin becomes thicker and tougher than that of women. Sebum output, which escalates in both sexes, is always higher in males. While this – together with those galloping hormones – means greasy faces, spots and acne for something like seven out of ten male teenagers, it also brings more life-long protection. While female sebum output is always lower and goes into a small but steady decline from puberty onwards and can drop drastically sometime in the forties, men's sebum output peaks at thirty, then drops a little, but stays fairly constant until well beyond middle age, and only drops dramatically in old age.

But be warned, it's never plain-sailing with skin. Stress, pollution, air travel, air conditioning, poor eating habits, alcohol, sun and weather extremes, and lack of fresh air and exercise can all dehydrate any skin. And to balance out any natural inbuilt wrinkle-proofing, men give their skins more daily wear and tear and, despite some recent improvements, less care.

A predeliction for diving into muddy playing fields, sweating profusely during various games and outdoor activities, and sunbathing without sunscreens and moisturisers, plus a high natural sensitivity to fragrance in after-shaves and soaps and the daily tussle with a beard can all contribute to balancing out gender advantages. So, take good care of yourself if you want to keep the wrinkles at bay, and your skin clean, soothed and free from rashes and dry, irritated patches.

Cleansing

Don't lather your face for washing with the nearest bar of soap. Male skins are particularly sensitive to fragrance; strong soap can strip the skin's natural protection and leave an irritating residue. Use a mild, non-perfumed soap or, better still, a cleansing bar or wash-off foaming cleanser.

Deep cleansing

Give your skin a regular weekly treatment with a facial scrub to remove dead skin cells and debris. Scrubs also help ingrown hairs to break free.

Professional salon treatments

A facial is luxurious and very good for deep cleansing the skin. Many beauty therapists give treatments to males these days, and there are salons exclusively for men. So, why not give yourself an occasional treat and be kind to your skin.

Face masks

If your skin is oily and prone to blackheads, choose a mask which is formulated to remove surface impurities. Older or dried-up skins will benefit from a moisturising mask.

Shaving cream or foam

Read the labels. Be wary of products that promise to soften the beard – they may also 'soften' the skin, and make it more prone to cuts and razor burn.

After shaves

Fragrance and alcohol – both found in many aftershaves – can be irritating to a skin already edgy after shaving. If you love the smell of yours, use it on your throat and shoulders, not on freshly sheared skin. Choose a non-alcoholic, fragrance-free, soothing balm or a non-perfumed moisturiser for post-shave faces.

Protection

Use a lightweight moisturiser to protect against dehydrating conditions, both indoors and out – one with UV filters will help prevent sun damage. When you're doing outdoor sports or lazing in the sun, always wear a high SPF sunscreen on your face. If your forehead's very high or you have a bald patch, use sunscreen on those areas. Scalps are particularly prone to burning.

Male superfluous hair

Eyebrows that beetle across the bridge of the nose look untidy but are very easy to get rid of. Find yourself a good electrolysist who will take male clients and get the superfluous hairs removed for good.

As men grow older, downy hairs on the ears, nose and cheeks can convert to coarser hair. Again, some electrolysists will treat these if they trouble you. Eyebrows have a tendency to beetle and sprout wildly. Some hairdressers will trim these or you can keep them in line yourself. Comb eyebrows upwards and carefully trim off hairs that sprout way beyond the upper line of your brows with a small pair of scissors. There is now a neat, battery-operated gadget for home use that will safely trim all this super-fluous hair.

SHAVING

The biggest difference between men and women's faces is the coarseness of hair. The daily tussle with a beard can end up being a skin endurance test if it's not done carefully and properly. If you've been shaving without tears for years, that's fine. But, if you have problems every morning, consider whether you could improve your shaving techniques.

The following hints will help you achieve a comfortable, close wet shave:

- before *wet shaving*, wash the face and leave the final warm rinsing water on the beard for two minutes – this causes the hair to expand about thirty-four per cent, making it softer and easier to cut

- apply a good lather of shaving cream or gel to prevent water evaporation and reduce friction between skin and blade

- use light strokes, and as few as possible in the direction of hair growth

- shave jawline, cheeks and neck first, chin and upper lip last – whiskers are tougher here, and need more time to absorb the water and shaving product

- rinse the razor frequently during shaving to get rid of debris

- finally, rinse your face with lukewarm water, pat dry with a towel and moisturise your skin

If you prefer power behind your cutting strokes:

- *electric shavers* work best against dry, hard beards. A pre-shave powder stick (like a stick of solid talc) will absorb oil or perspiration and help the shaver to glide more smoothly over the skin. A specially formulated pre-electric lotion will lubricate the skin, reduce friction, and stiffen the beard, but will evaporate quickly leaving it dry

- use short strokes and little pressure. For problem areas, stretch the skin taut and try a circular motion with the shaver

- use the trimmer on any longer hairs, and on moustaches and sideburns

- finally, remember always to moisturise skin, and clean the razor blades.

Off with his beard

Research by Remington and Gillette highlight some beard facts and man's timeless battle with whiskers . . .

- a man's beard grows an average of one fifteen thousandth of an inch a day or 5½ inches a year . . . it covers about one third of a square foot and contains 15,500 hairs – give or take a hair or two

- the average wet shaver will spend about seventy hours a year removing the whiskers from his face

- dry beard hair is about as tough as copper wire of the same thickness

- you will get a closer shave when you've been up for half an hour or so. Your face is puffy when you first fall out of bed

- changing your razor? Give it time – it takes 4 weeks or so for you and your face to get used to a new shaver.

A brief history of shaving

Bronze age man shaved, and was often buried with shavers and tweezers. Priests and higher classes in Ancient Egypt shaved their whole bodies. Noble Romans doused themselves with oil and shaved on Tuesdays. Alexander the Great insisted on his warriors shaving daily so the enemy had nothing to grab hold of in hand-to-hand fighting. Peter the Great of Russia gave his male subjects a choice – either shave or have your beard pulled out bristle by bristle. Jean Jacques Perret invented the first known safety razor in 1750 after catching a skin disease in one of the often unhygienic barber shops. Beards and barber shops still flourished until two major happenings changed the face of man. Gillette invented a throwaway blade for safety razors in 1902 (until then safety razors had to be 'stropped' or sharpened to keep the blade sharp) and at the outbreak of the First World War every soldier in the British and American armies was issued with a razor and ordered to shave for self-preservation purposes – a gas mask on a bearded face was almost useless. Jacob Schick brought the first electric shaver onto the market in 1931. Today about thirty per cent of men use electric shavers and around seventy per cent wet shave. A battery operated wet razor has recently been introduced onto the market.

(History of shaving courtesy of Remington Consumer Products)

CHAPTER FOUR

LOOK AFTER YOUR BODY

HEALTHY EATING

Of course, no-one can promise you a flawless skin through eating 'healthy' foods and yes, we all seem to know someone who stuffs themselves on chocolate, chips and rubbish foods and seems to thrive. But generally, the eating plan for good health and a good skin is the same – a sensible, well-balanced diet based on a wide variety of fresh food – a diet high in fibre, generous in unrefined carbohydrates, adequate in protein and low in fat with little or no added sugar or salt; a diet which provides all the vitamins and minerals your body needs to function at its best.

The food group with the biggest part to play in the formation and functioning of healthy skin is protein. Like all body tissue, skin is made from protein – or, more correctly, from a combination of amino acids derived from the protein you eat. Just as the process of skin renewal is continuous, the need for protein is continuous too – though an adult's requirement is less than that of a growing child.

Fats and unrefined carbohydrate foods are also essential for skin health, not least because – along with protein – they supply the vitamins and minerals which are essential for the efficient running of your body system. Your skin particularly needs vitamins A and C as well as several from the B group, plus zinc. It's best to get the vitamins you need from a balanced diet, although deficiencies can be offset with supplements. Cellulose carbohydrates, better known as fibre foods, have another, less direct effect on the skin. Their action in keeping you 'regular' can help to give you a brighter and clearer complexion.

The most essential element in your diet – water – is also partly provided by the foods you eat, but it's important that you also drink at least 1 litre of water or other beverages a day to keep your body hydrated.

Big weight fluctuations are disastrous for your body and your skin. Regularly eating more than you need thickens the subcutaneous fat layer and stretches the elastic fibres of the dermis. Stay that way and you'll be overweight (with all the aesthetic and health problems that accompany this), but your skin will probably be plumped out. The trouble is that overweight people usually make mighty attempts to lose excess weight from time to time and when the pounds roll off too fast this can lead to skin 'collapse', leaving them with lines, sags and wrinkles. Drastic diets that are followed for any length of time are also likely to leave you short of essential nutrients, with consequent disadvantages for your skin. A sensible diet, which lets you slim slowly if you're overweight or keeps your weight on an even keel if you're not, combined with regular exercise and moisturising will keep your face and body looking fit and youthful in every way.

So what is a sensible eating pattern that will keep you healthy, in good shape and doing your best by your skin? Consultant nutritionist and dietician Jane Griffin has provided the guidelines in the Healthy Eating Plan on pages 64–5.

Of course, you can vary your meals much more than this outline suggests, with occasional restaurant meals, cooked breakfasts, pizza, made-up pasta dishes, soups, stews and casseroles, as well as cooked desserts based on fruit. But try to follow these basic rules:

- Eat as wide a variety of foods as you can, including some each day from all the food groups given in the outline.

- Eat some fruit and vegetables *raw* and try to have a salad every day.

- Cook vegetables lightly, preferably by steaming them. If you do boil them, use little water, and save the water for soups, sauces or gravies.

- To conserve vitamins, don't prepare vegetables too long before you cook or serve them, do keep their skins on whenever possible, and don't overcook them or keep them warm for a long time after cooking.

- Choose brown rice, wholemeal bread, cereals and pasta whenever possible.

- Replace some of the animal protein in your diet (ie meat, poultry, fish, cheese and eggs) with vegetable protein – cereals, nuts, pulses (ie peas, beans and lentils).

- Base your meals on their fibre and carbohydrate content and start to regard the protein as a smaller 'side' dish.

- Cut down on fat by switching to low-fat milk, cheeses and spreads and by grilling instead of frying foods or baking instead of roasting them.

- Avoid pastry, pies, fatty processed meat and solid fats (like lard and block margarine) and cut down on hard cheeses, cream and ice cream.

- Skim fat from soups and casseroles.

- Cut out cakes, biscuits, sweets and chocolates, except for a very occasional treat.

- Switch to low-calorie mayonnaise and salad dressing if you use these products regularly and look for low-calorie versions of bought salads.

- Don't add sugar to coffee or tea – if you can't do without sweetening, use a sweetener instead.

- Cut out soft, sugary drinks and have fruit juice or water instead.

- Cut out spirits, but you may have two glasses of wine with your main meal 3 or 4 times a week.

- If you eat tinned fruit from time to time, look for sugar-free varieties in fruit juice not syrup.

- Don't add salt to foods served at the table and use much less or none at all in cooking.

- Avoid salty snack foods like crisps and salted nuts.

- Cut down on sauces and pickles which have a high salt content.

- Avoid processed foods which have added salt and – sometimes – sugar, check labels of canned foods for these additives, too.

- Always remember that 'Fresh is best!'

- Don't eat 'on the run'. Make time for your meals, and be relaxed when you eat them – that way you'll eat more slowly, know when you've had enough and feel fuller and more satisfied.

- Don't despair if you sometimes stray from the nutritional straight and narrow. Occasional sweets and treats won't hurt any more than the occasional extra glass of wine. In fact, if either takes the edge off anxiety at the time, then what they do in lowering your stress level could offset the degree by which they raise your calorie intake or upset your healthy eating plan.

Your Healthy Eating Plan

Breakfast

Make a point of having a good breakfast, as you may not have eaten for the last 10–12 hours and your blood sugar is probably low which can lead to irritability, listlessness and poor performance. Your system can make more efficient use of this meal than any other.

Menu

fresh fruit or unsweetened fruit juice
(*note:* fruit has more fibre content than juice)
and porridge, unsweetened muesli, wheat or bran cereal
   (*note:* no sugar – for sweetness add fresh or dried fruit)
with semi-skimmed milk
and/or wholemeal bread or toast
with low-fat spread
and reduced-sugar marmalade or jam, peanut butter, mashed banana, cottage cheese or lean ham

Main meal

Ideally, have this in the middle of the day, again because your system can then make more efficient use of the calories it contains.

Menu

lean meat, fish or poultry (3–4 times a week)
eggs and/or cheese (1–2 times a week)
beans, pulses or nuts (1–2 times a week)
with potato (ideally cooked in its skin)
or brown rice
or wholemeal pasta
and 2–3 vegetables, lightly cooked
(vary your choice, and include green, yellow or orange vegetables frequently.)
then fresh fruit
or yoghurt

Light meal

Ideally, have this in the evening, but if you go out to work or prefer to eat your main meal at night, make this meal your lunch. Try not to eat your last meal late at night:

Menu

wholemeal bread sandwich, 2–4 slices with peanut butter
or low-fat cheese
or lean meat
or poultry
or fish (choose oily fish twice a week)
and a large salad of raw, mixed vegetables
then fresh fruit
or yoghurt

Throughout the day

Drink plenty of water, unsweetened fruit juices and moderate amounts of tea and/or coffee – no sugar – with semi-skimmed milk, or black. Ideally, choose herbal or decaffeinated tea and decaffeinated coffee.

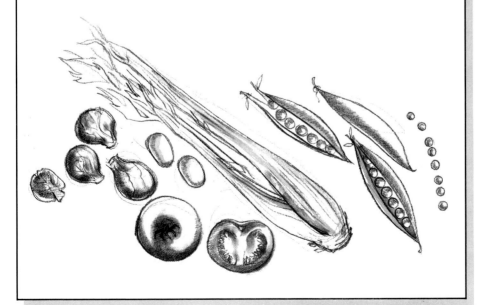

THE REFRESHER COURSE

As the daily food plan has shown, a variety of fresh foods is the best recipe for all-round health. But not every food agrees with everybody, and this conflict often shows up on the skin. If you suspect that your skin problems could be related to what you eat, try Jane Griffin's Refresher Course opposite. It will certainly help you to brighter, clearer skin and may also help to pinpoint problem foods for you.

VITAMINS, MINERALS AND SUPPLEMENTARY BENEFITS

The 'vita' in vitamins means *life* and these micro-nutrients are certainly vital to life, health and lasting looks. Although they have no direct energy value or body-building function, they play an essential role in the chain link that regulates our metabolic processes, converts carbohydrates and fats into energy, forms bone and tissue and generally keeps mind and body functioning at optimum level.

Vitamins fall into two groups; the fat-soluble A, D, E, F and K (usually measured in International Units – IU) which can be stored in the body, and the water-soluble B complex, C and P (measured in milligrammes, or mg) which cannot be stored in the body, so any excess goes down the lavatory each day.

Taking supplementary vitamins and minerals is a controversial issue. Most nutritionists and medical people say it's unnecessary (except in special cases such as children, pregnant women, certain medical conditions) and believe we get all we need from a healthy, well-balanced and varied diet. At the opposite extreme are the enthusiasts who feel no-one can function at optimum level without a handful of supplements.

I prefer the happy in-between suggested by clinical biochemist Leonard Mervyn, technical director of a major health food company. He is also a respected author of many books and research papers on the subject and a person who puts simple good sense into the subject, agreeing that in a perfect world we would get all the nutrients we need from our diet. *But*, as he says, how many of us can pick, cut or dig our own fruit, salad and vegetables? How long have the ones we buy been travelling or sitting on a shelf with strip lighting leaching what's left of their original goodness?

Much shopping is done in a supermarket swoop for the sake of convenience, so foodstuffs languish in the fridge for days before they get to our

The Refresher Course

Days 1 and 2

Eat only fresh fruits and vegetables. Choose any six of the following fruits:

apples	grapes	pineapple	cherries	raspberries
apricots	nectarines	plums	pears	strawberries
bananas	peaches	oranges	grapefruit	

Have at least 8 oz/250 g of fresh salad dressed with olive oil and lemon juice, at any one or two meals, made from at least six of the following:

lettuce	celery	parsley	carrot
tomatoes	cucumber	peppers	radishes
beetroot	cauliflower	mushrooms	watercress

Eat at least one jacket-baked potato, minimum weight 6 oz/150 g plus as much of as many other steamed vegetables as you wish.

Eat as many meals as you wish, whenever it suits you. Have fruit for breakfast and as mid-morning and mid-afternoon snacks. Eat potatoes and hot vegetables plus fruit for your midday meal, and an 8 oz/250 g raw mixed salad followed by fruit for your evening meal.

Days 3 and 4

Introduce wholegrains. Have bread or toast if you wish. Add muesli or another cereal, served with fruit juice instead of milk, for breakfast. Avoid dairy foods on these two days. Don't spread butter on your bread, but use vegetable-based margarine. Keep up the water intake. Drink moderate amounts of fruit juice and herb or lemon tea on the first six days of this refresher course.

Days 5 and 6

Introduce fish, meat and poultry. Choose fresh – no tinned or processed foods at this time. Grill, bake, poach or steam foods.

Day 7

Introduce dairy foods – milk, cheese, eggs

Note: This seven day body refreshing food plan can be followed two or three times a year. True exclusion diets, which pinpoint food allergies, should be conducted over a longer period and only under close medical supervision. This course can only give a general indication of foods which you may tolerate less well than others.

plates. Your pint of milk will have lost most of its nutrients if it's been left on a sunny doorstep for a couple of hours, and your frozen vegetables much of theirs (in their thawed water) if you don't cook them straight from the freezer. Poor cooking methods, over-processed and over-refined foods, eating out (when we don't know how long the food has been sitting and steaming), pesticides, pollution in the atmosphere, illness and stress in our lives, medicinal drugs, contraceptive pills, habits like smoking cigarettes and drinking alcohol can either destroy vitamins and minerals or increase our body's requirements.

So do your best to follow a nutritionally sound diet, check the food source chart to see you're on to the right foodstuffs, and follow the buying and preparation tips to prove you're not wasting nutrients. Then add a daily dose of Leonard Mervyn's suggested health 'insurance policy' supplement, of one high potency multi-vitamin and mineral capsule or pill (which should give you safe coverage of all you need). Read the amounts given on the labels and make sure they contain 400IU vitamin E, 400IU vitamin D, and 15mg zinc. If not, top up to the required amount with other supplements.

Those who indulge in hard sports (eg squash) or long-term ones (eg marathons) should augment their mineral intake, because significant amounts can be lost in sweat.

Women who suffer from pre-menstrual problems can take 25–100mg vitamin B6 daily for a week or more before a period, which should ease the symptoms. Leonard Mervyn advises that the contraceptive pill can induce deficiency of certain vitamins and minerals, particularly B_2, B_6, B_{12}, folic acid, biotin, vitamin C, manganese and zinc, so supplements of them (or a

---

Megavitamin therapy

In the past thirty years the use of *clinically controlled* megavitamin therapy has grown. Vitamin B complex is now used in the treatment of some mental diseases; vitamin E for heart and circulatory problems; vitamin C for its anti-infective properties; vitamins A and C for burns; vitamin A for certain skin conditions. The response has often been dramatic, and even with massive doses side effects were virtually non-existent except sometimes in the cases of vitamins A and D and these disappeared when the dose was reduced.

good 'all-round' supplement containing all these vitamins and minerals) can help reduce some of the side-effects of the Pill.

For the older person (60 and above), extra *Choline* (loosely regarded as a B vitamin, but not a true one), can help overcome forgetfulness and mental vagueness. The best way to take high dose choline is as lecithin, which, because it is rich in essential fatty acids will also benefit the skin. There is strong evidence to suggest that it is important to build up strong bones by taking extra calcium and magnesium before and during the menopause rather than after it when osteoporosis may set in. Even then, extra calcium can slow down progression of the condition.

VITAMINS – WHAT THEY DO FOR YOU

Vitamin A
Rich food sources of this crucial vitamin are cod liver oil, halibut liver oil, liver, butter, cheese, eggs, milk. Can be taken as beta-carotene in carrots, green vegetables, tomatoes, asparagus, apricots, peaches, melons. Vitamin A is vital to your sight, it's important if you want to 'see in the dark' or if you work with VDUs. It also helps maintain healthy skin, bones and teeth, and builds resistance to infection. Deficiency can lead to dry, scaly skin, susceptibility to skin infections, rough 'goose flesh', and night blindness. Destroyed by light, high temperatures, iron and copper pans.

Vitamin B₁ (thiamine)
A member of the vitamin B complex. Rich sources of this vitamin are yeast, wholegrains, meat, offal, and green vegatables. Most foods contain some, but it's easily destroyed by heat, alkali (eg baking powder), and lost in thawing drips. Vitamin B_1 converts carbohydrate into energy in the muscles and nervous system. Deficiency can cause fatigue, nausea, muscle weakness, and digestive problems. Requirements will be increased during pregnancy, when breast feeding, or under stress. The elderly also need extra.

Vitamin B₂ (riboflavin)
A member of the vitamin B complex. Rich sources of this vitamin are yeast, liver, wheatgerm, cheese, eggs, milk, green leafy vegetables, pulses. Vitamin B_2 assists in the production and repair of body tissues. Deficiency leads to cracks and sores at corners of mouth, scaly skin, itchy eyes, hair loss and mouth ulcers. Extra may be needed by drinkers, smokers, and women on the contraceptive pill.

Vitamin B_6 (pyridoxine)

A member of the vitamin B complex. Rich sources of this vitamin are yeast, wholegrains, nuts, meat, fish, potatoes, green leaf and root vegetables, eggs, bananas and dried fruits. Vitamin B_6 is the anti-depressant vitamin – it helps regulate the nervous system. It may be used to treat PMS, morning sickness, travel sickness, and depression induced by the Pill. Deficiency may lead to skin complaints, mild depression, premenstrual problems, infantile convulsions and heart problems.

Vitamin B_{12} (cobalamin)

A member of the vitamin B complex. Rich sources of this vitamin are offal, meat, fish, eggs, poultry, cheese, yoghurt, and milk. Vitamin B_{12} is an essential element in normal cell division, maintaining the energy reserve in muscles, and nerve fibre insulation. Deficiency in B_{12} can lead to nervous and menstrual disorders, and severe deficiency can lead to pernicious anaemia. Animal sources mean vegans can have problems, but it is now possible to obtain B_{12} from a mould fermentation (non-animal source), (enquire at your local health shop).

Biotin

A member of the vitamin B complex. Rich sources of this vitamin are yeast, offal, eggs, wholegrains, fish, meat, milk, cheese, yoghurt. (Biotin is also produced by intestinal bacteria.) Biotin is involved in many metabolic processes and is essential for maintenance of healthy skin, hair, and the regulation of sex hormones.

Folic acid

A member of the vitamin B complex. Rich sources of this vitamin are yeast, wholegrains, nuts, offal, citrus fruits, eggs, fish, green leaf and root vegetables, cheese, meat, milk, pulses. Folic acid is essential for protein synthesis and production of normal red blood cells. Deficiency can lead to megaloblastic anaemia where blood cells change shape and size and have a shorter life span. Functions with vitamin B_{12} in blood formation.

Niacin

A member of the vitamin B complex. Rich sources of this vitamin are yeast, wholegrains, chicken, nuts, liver, fish, cheese, eggs, pulses. Niacin assists in the breakdown and utilisation of fats, protein and carbohydrates. Helps maintain healthy brain, nerves, skin and digestive organs. Severe deficiency is responsible for *pellagra* (Italian for rough skin) which progresses from dermatitis, diarrhoea and dementia to death.

Pantothenic acid

This is a member of the vitamin B complex. Rich sources of this vitamin are yeast, offal, nuts, wholegrains, meat, eggs, poultry, pulses, leaf and root vegetables, cheese, yoghurt and fruits. Pantothenic acid is known as the anti-stress vitamin, because it makes for a healthy nervous system. May reduce adverse effects of antibiotics. It has been used therapeutically to decrease allergic skin reactions in children and to relieve morning stiffness in arthritis.

Vitamin C (ascorbic acid)

Rich sources of this vitamin are most fruit and vegetables. Vitamin C plays a strong part in manufacture of collagen, strong capillaries and resistance to bacterial and viral diseases. It helps any type of wound healing process. Deficiency leads to slow healing, bruising, bleeding gums, weakness, and lassitude. Great deficiency leads to scurvy – the scourge of old-time sailors, which was remedied by taking fruit and vegetables on long voyages. Vitamin C is easily lost in cooking. More will be needed after injury, during infection, when taking antibiotics, by the elderly, athletes, smokers, alcohol drinkers and women on the Pill.

Vitamin C tablets

Colds and hangovers are hard on looks, dry out your skin, and make you unlively and unlovely. Try these remedies and you could save yourself unnecessary suffering:

- Vitamin C supplements to combat or cure colds is another controversial issue, but this works wonders for me and everyone I've suggested it to. When you're nursing the sort of cold that makes your limbs feel as though they belong to someone else and your skin like sore sandpaper, try taking 500 mg vitamin C (with orange juice or water) each hour for five hours (1 × 500mg). At least you'll look and feel half human the next day.

- If you've dined and wined too well and know you're going to regret it the next day, take 500mg vitamin C just before going to bed, and another 500mg first thing in the morning as soon as you wake up. You'll hardly know you over-indulged on alcohol.

Vitamin D

Rich sources of this vitamin are cod liver oil, oily fish, tinned fish – salmon, mackerel, sardines, tuna – dairy products and eggs. Significant amounts produced by sunlight on the skin. Vitamin D has a prime role in bone formation. Deficiency leads to rickets and osteomalacia (an adult form of rickets) which are both characterised by softening of the bones. Toxicity has been found when doses of 10,000IU were taken daily over a long period of time. As 400IU is the recommended daily limit without prescription, there is little likelihood of running into any trouble.

Vitamin E

Rich sources of this vitamin are vegetable and fish oils, shellfish, liver, brown rice, potatoes, most fruits and vegetables. Vitamin E is an anti-blood-clotting agent. It strengthens capillary walls, neutralises the effect of harmful free radicals, counteracts premature ageing and helps generate new skin. Increased intakes have been found helpful in aiding healing after burns, diminishing menopausal symptoms such as flushing, depression, panic attacks. It is used also for circulatory problems. Deficiency of vitamin E can cause premature ageing, lack of vitality, disinterest in physical and sexual activity.

MINERALS – WHAT THEY DO FOR YOU

Minerals are the essential little co-workers that keep your body functioning smoothly by acting as catalysts in bio-chemical reactions as well as in structural, nerve-transmission and oxygen-carrying roles. Although quantities of some are minute (so minute they're called trace minerals), there's hardly a process they don't affect, from preserving the health of heart, brain and nerve transmission system, through structural functions – bones, teeth, soft tissue – to influencing glandular performance and controlling the body's fluid balance. Minerals act as a buffer to neutralise toxic and harmful substances inside and outside the body (stress, atmospheric pollution, highly acid or alkaline foods) and they play a vital role in hair and skin health.

Calcium

Good sources of calcium are dairy products, green vegetables, fish (particularly canned fish with softened bones), wholegrains and fortified bread. Works with vitamin D looking after health of bones, teeth, heart, muscles, nervous system; with vitamin A to keep skin healthy.

Chlorine
Good sources of chlorine are green leaf vegetables, tomatoes, salt. Usually obtained with sodium and potassium – a major aid to digestive processes and absorption of nutrients.

Cobalt
Good sources of cobalt are green leaf vegetables, fruit, wholegrains. Cobalt is a trace mineral that only functions as part of vitamin B_{12}.

Copper
Good sources of copper are poultry, offal, shellfish, green leafy vegetables, wholegrains, nuts. Copper works with iron in production of red blood cells. Important for health of muscle, skin and nerve fibres.

Fluorine
Good sources of fluorine are seafood, tea, some drinking water. Fluorine strengthens teeth and bones, reduces incidence of dental caries and possibly osteoporosis.

Iodine
Good sources of iodine are any food from the sea or food that is grown near the sea. Iodine is a trace element that's involved with smooth functioning of the thyroid gland – the pacemaker for metabolic activities of the body.

Iron
Good sources of iron are meat, offal, shellfish, green vegetables, wholegrains, soya beans, potatoes, egg yolks, sunflower seeds. Iron works together with vitamin C and is involved in the formation of haemoglobin and transportation of oxygen to muscle tissue. Iron is lost during menstruation/childbirth and extra may be prescribed during pregnancy or for habitually heavy periods.

Magnesium
Good sources of magnesium are green vegetables, seafood, pulses. It is present in most foods and is necessary for the metabolism of calcium and vitamin D. Magnesium is essential to life, as it helps keep muscles, bones, nerves and heart functioning well.

Phosphorus
Good sources of phosphorus are most foods, especially dairy products, fish, wholegrains. Phosphorus is found in nearly every part of the body,

and it is important for growth, maintenance of cells and all aspects of energy production and utilisation.

Potassium

Good sources are citrus fruits, pulses, potatoes, green leaf vegetables, seafood, tomatoes, avocados, bananas, and dried fruits. Also see sodium.

Sodium

Good sources of sodium are salt and salted foods (bacon etc), seafood and green vegetables. Sodium and potassium work together to regulate fluid balance in the body.

Selenium

Good sources of selenium are offal, seafood, wholegrains and nuts. Selenium works with vitamin E to neutralise the effect of free radicals and retard the ageing process and it increases the ability of white blood cells to resist infection.

Sulphur

Good sources of sulphur are dairy products, chicken, fish, meat, pulses and nuts. It is present in thiamine and biotin (B complex vitamins) and in essential amino acids. It helps in the formation of body tissues and plays an important part in keeping skin in good order.

Zinc

Good sources of zinc are meat, wholegrains, milk, pulses, and nuts. Zinc is vital for the metabolism of vitamin A. It has an essential role in the body's enzyme systems, cell growth, tissue repair, gland functions, skin health, healing and the immune system.

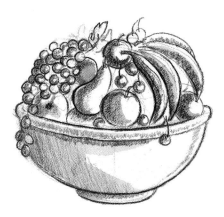

CONSERVING VITAMINS AND MINERALS IN FOOD

The way you buy, prepare and cook your vegetables can save or squander so much of their vitamin and mineral content as well as their taste. Try to follow these guidelines to get the best out of what you eat:

- Avoid using processed foods except as an occasional source of convenience. Choose the freshest foods possible, eat as many salads, fresh vegetables and unrefined foods as you can. Make soups and casseroles when the weather's cold – it's not always psychologically sound to eat cold, damp food on a cold, damp day.

- Plant your patch if you have one (and if you're well outside cities and away from pollution) with some salads and vegetables. Many will grow in a small space, share the plot with flowers, grow up walls and fences. If you live without a garden, investigate bean and grain sprouting which will only take up a small corner of the kitchen, bring in a good source of vitamins, and are fast and fun to grow.

- Shop daily for vegetables. If you can't, store them in an airy, cool, dark place or in the fridge.

- Prepare vegetables just before you're going to cook and eat them. Avoid peeling – vitamins and minerals congregate under the peel and the fibre is good for you. Because of chemical sprays and pesticides, always wash your fruit and vegetables thoroughly and if you have any choice in the matter opt for fruit and vegetables that have not been sprayed. Remove peel after cooking if you must. Cook whole or cut in large pieces and keep leaves whole to avoid losing nutrients by exposure to air.

- Steam or pressure cook when you can, so food is over rather than in the water. Otherwise, put vegetables into boiling water, use the minimum amount of water and cook for the shortest possible time. Save the water for soups, casseroles and gravies or drink it straight. Never add bicarbonate of soda which destroys vitamin C and thiamine. Add salt at the end of cooking if you must take it.

- Cook frozen vegetables straight from the freezer. If there's some hold-up, put them in a container while they wait for the pot, so any thawed liquid is added to the cooking (it's full of vitamins).

- Copper and iron cooking utensils can destroy some vitamins. Go for stainless steel, glass or enamel. Serve as soon as cooked. Keeping food warm will destroy a lot of the nutrients.

OTHER VALUABLE SUPPLEMENTS

Fish oils

Cod liver oil was prescribed by British doctors in the eighteenth century for people suffering from bone disease and rheumatism. The Victorians used it for treating infections, nervous illness and skin diseases. The only thing that has changed is that today's medical profession now understands more about just how it works.

Apart from being one of the richest sources of vitamins A and D, fish body and fish liver oils contain two polyunsaturated fatty acids – EPA and DHA – which have been found to reduce blood fat levels and blood clotting and so reduce the risk of heart disease and strokes. Fish oil concentrate can improve the symptoms of rheumatoid arthritis and other inflammatory disorders including eczema and psoriasis. Its role in promoting growth, strong bones, well-behaved skin and building resistance to infection is as accepted now as it was in Victorian times.

Fish oil supplements can be taken as oil or capsules and the addition of malt extract or orange syrup makes them acceptable to children's taste.

Garlic

The bulb of this pungent plant is widely used for flavouring meat, fish, vegetables and salads. It has also been valued for thousands of years as a medicine and antiseptic. It was highly prized for its medicinal qualities in Ancient Greece and Egypt and the Romans used it to treat coughs, colds, lung diseases and wounds.

Nearer our own times, the military re-discovered its healing properties and it was used on wounds during the First World War and about the same time for the treatment of tuberculosis in hospitals. In the 1950s scientific proof backed all those years of faith in its properties when it was discovered that garlic contained *allicin*, which is a powerful antibacterial agent. Today its helping us to cope with 'modern' diseases. It has been found that garlic helps to lower high blood pressure and cholesterol levels – providing protection against the risk of strokes and heart disease. Garlic also stimulates the digestive system and inhibits retention of waste substances in the body.

Used externally, there were many old country remedies based on garlic for digestive, bronchial, rheumatic and complexion problems. (A screw-topped jar filled with garlic cloves steeped for a week in boiled cider vinegar is reputed to produce a garlic vinegar that, when dabbed on spots, helps to clear them, but I haven't tried this remedy!)

If you don't like the taste of garlic or the anti-social side of its after-affects on the breath, you can buy capsules of deodorised garlic or coated tables which still contain allicin, the potent part. The coating doesn't melt until the tablet is well on its way into the digestive system, thus reducing any risks of garlic-laden breath.

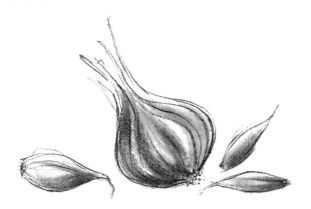

Oil of evening primrose

The oil extracted from the seeds of the Evening Primrose has hit the headlines in the past few years due to its apparent abilities to help in so many major and minor body breakdowns.

Native to Central America, where it was used for healing, the plant's seeds found their way into ships' cargoes in the eighteenth century, and the plant became naturalised in Europe, growing wild in the countryside.

The seed oil is unique in that it contains substantial amounts of gamma-linolenic acid (GLA) which is converted in the body to substances which help in the growth and reproduction of cells. GLA is produced in the body from dietary linoleic acid, but it seems that synthesis can sometimes be blocked or not sufficient for the body's needs.

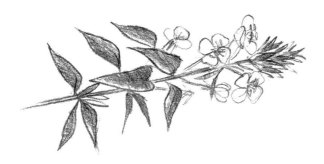

Oil of Evening Primrose has been used with success in treating such diverse conditions as eczema, psoriasis, pre-menstrual and menopausal problems, hyperactivity in children, arthritis and other inflammatory conditions, disorders of the immune system, alcoholism, and multiple sclerosis. There is no toxicity and usual intakes are 3 to 6 capsules a day (each capsule providing 500mg oil). Externally the oil, on its own or contained in creams and lotions, is used as a moisturiser.

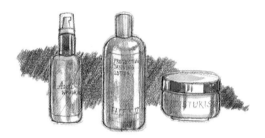

EXERCISE AND RELAXATION

You can spend a minor fortune on skin care products, and lavish time, care and meticulous attention on the surface, but the all-important renewal process of your skin starts from the inside. Armed for life with a sound eating programme, you're on your way. Now get the rest of your body-enhancing plans into focus and give your skin a sound start.

EXERCISE

Exercise encourages the circulation to zip around, supplying nourishment to all parts of the body. It increases energy, encourages relaxation and sound sleep, and tones up your muscles giving your skin a sound sub-structure. And it does great things for your mind as well as your body, releasing hormone-like substances – the natural 'happy drugs' – that help you throw off mild depression and frustration. Above all, exercise can be fun. It can make you feel confident, happy with your body and with yourself.

If it's many years since you've made your body move around a lot, start gently, so it's given time to adapt to the increased demand for oxygen and the extra work given to muscles. Choose the type of exercise that's right for you and your lifestyle. Ideally, it should increase your suppleness, strength and stamina without adding stress to your life.

The easiest, cheapest and most relaxing exercise is walking, as long as you're not bowed down with bags (consider a rucksack if you constantly have a lot to carry – it's better for your posture). Why not leave the car in the garage, let the bus go by and take on some daily mileage in the fresh air? Stride out with arms swinging – you can speed up to a gentle jog providing you're wearing proper running shoes to prevent joint jolt.

Try swimming – it can't be said often enough that it's *the* best all-round exercise. Also try cycling if you won't be overcome with traffic fumes and tension. Games are a good idea, if you find competition stimulating. Join a nearby keep fit class – anything from stretch and stamina sessions to yoga, a touch of tap dancing or working with light weights.

Little and often is far better than a hectic hour or more once a week. If time, money, or lack of facilities make organised exercise difficult, keep on walking and work out some top-to-toe stretches that take no more than fifteen minutes a day to do at home. Try to get a friend or the whole family going. Like most things, it's more fun with a companion.

As regards the skin you can see, leave off make-up when you exercise for any length of time. Do use a moisturiser, or a sunscreen if you're leaping around outside in the sun.

POSTURE

Good posture helps you to look and feel vital. Bad posture is a physical and mental burden that hampers your breathing capacity and adds tension to your body – a badly held spine and unbalanced body will bring you pain and worn out body parts sooner rather than later. Hold your body well and you're literally standing up for yourself and persuading others of your positive, confident attitude to life.

Good posture is upright but relaxed, not 'guards officer' stiff. Lift and lengthen your spine and keep your neck long as though an invisible wire attached to the crown of your head was lifting you to the ceiling. Hold the chin at right angles to the ground, not out, up, or tucked in. Shoulders should be back and down – find their proper natural place by lifting your shoulders an inch or two, pulling them back and then letting them relax down, so shoulder blades and muscles move towards the spine and your arms hang loosely at your sides. When you're standing, keep feet hip-width apart so they give your body a firm base and keep your weight evenly balanced over the entire foot.

Walk by placing your heel down first, and 'peeling' the feet off the ground, so you work through the entire foot to the toes and put a bounce in your step.

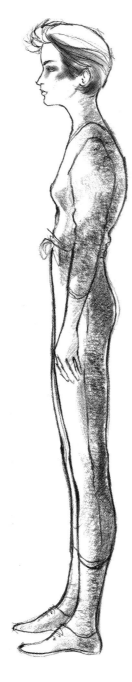

Standing badly

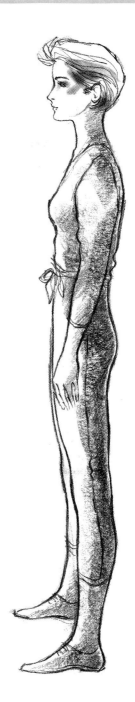

Standing properly

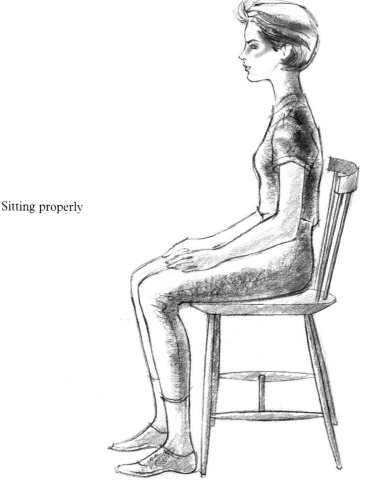

Sitting properly

When you take the weight off your feet, choose an upright chair with a firm back and sit well back in it with your feet firmly on the floor and slightly apart. Televisions should be positioned high enough for you to view in comfort without slouching. And remember to take your new-found good posture to bed with you, with a firm, comfortable mattress and a pillow that supports your neck without throwing your head in the air and encouraging chin sags and a bent spine.

BREATHING

From our first cry to our final farewell, breathing is an all-time essential – without oxygen our life can be measured in minutes. Yet we waste this potential health and beauty maker by taking quick gasps of air, using only part of our lungs and rarely clearing them. Shallow breathing adversely affects our energy levels, endurance and concentration capacities and it can lead to a variety of disorders from respiratory tract infections to skin problems and nervous tension.

Learn to retrain your lungs and get them back to full working capacity. As you inhale through your nose, aim that intake down into the region of your stomach (your abdomen will balloon out a little) which fills the lower part of your lungs. Pull your stomach in and continue that intake of air so your ribcage expands sideways, and the top of your chest lifts as the lungs fill. Hold the breath for a few seconds, then exhale fully by breathing out through your mouth (this allows you a more complete exhalation). Wait a few seconds and repeat. Do several sessions a day to begin with and soon you'll be into better breathing habits without conscious thought or effort.

STRESS

Stress receives very bad publicity, so let's get it into perspective now. It's the stuff that gets deeds done – without it we are cabbage-like, dull and unproductive. You can have a high-powered job, a houseful of children, and frequent heart-in-mouth situations, but if you love your life and can control the highs and hassle, you can cope with anything for any length of time. But, when stress becomes a strain, your mind and body don't enjoy the pressures and you can never get away from your worries, you're heading for a chronic state that affects your life, your health, and of course your looks, with tension lines around the eyes, mouth and on the forehead and a puffy, pasty or yellow skin that lacks the glow of life.

In primitive man, the source of stress called for a physical response. This was usually a run from danger or a fight for food. Heart, lungs, muscles and nervous system went on red alert, the immune and digestive system slowed down or stopped, surface blood vessels constricted as the flow was diverted to muscles, the skin turned pale and perspiration was released onto it to prepare for cooling after a heated effort. Back in the safety of his cave, happy he'd escaped or eaten his fill, primitive man had used physical energy to deal with a stressful situation; he'd resolved his problems and could sit back and relax.

In modern society our bodies react just as they did in primitive man, but problems can rarely be resolved in a physical way. How often can you run away from a depressing situation? Can you really beat up an impossible boss or that man who crashed into your car and get it all out of your system? Yet your body has gone through the fight or flight reaction and become all wound up with no means of physical release.

When the situation continues over long periods, the body revolts at its constantly unbalanced state. From poor sleep patterns, digestive disorders, a spate of bad colds and general lethargy, it can progress to serious physical and mental illness. Medically prescribed drugs can cloak the symptoms. They don't solve the problems. Only you can do that by quietly sitting down and working out what you can change in your life and how you can cope with situations you can't change.

Try to control anger and frustration. The world is full of injustice – from the difficult neighbour or boss to the inhuman conditions suffered by people in many parts of the world. You must decide if you can do anything about any of it. If you can't, you will not do any good by worrying or getting angry about personal or global problems. Anger is a great source of stress to everyone. Let it out and you hurt others. Keep it in and you hurt yourself.

A nutritionally sound diet, regular exercise, good posture and better breathing help your body with that task. Add the ability to unwind and you've almost beaten the modern malady.

RELAXATION

Everyone needs to 'shut off' now and again – how you manage it is a very personal matter. If a ten minute snooze restores and relaxes you, make sure you take it. Music can soothe many a frazzled nervous system. Or you can invest in one of the discs or tapes that have been specially developed to encourage relaxation and peace of mind. You know the way your mind and body work, so choose the way that suits *you*. One person revives after a quiet time, another needs a run round the block or time to indulge in a dearly loved hobby.

It doesn't matter what helps you to switch off, but it is important to find time to practise active relaxation for at least twenty minutes every day.

Meditation quietens the mind and produces a tranquillity that can stay with you throughout the day. There are several different methods involving breathing techniques, word repetition and body concentration. Self-hypnosis – with or without the use of tapes – and colour therapy (which involves self-hypnosis and colour visualising) can be wonderfully regenerative.

Yoga, with its quietly-held poses, breathing and relaxation techniques, provides both physical and mental release. It's the perfect means to slim, tone and balance your body and improve your ability to resist stress.

These methods of letting go need expert instruction in the techniques, so make some enquiries in your area.

Yoga relaxation

At home, try the yoga relaxation pose and see for yourself how it will clear your mind and increase your energy levels:

1. Lie on the floor if possible – a bed if you must – with your feet about 45cm apart and gently falling outwards, arms straight, palms facing upwards and a little away from your sides. Make sure your body is straight and symmetrical, and the top of your chin is more or less parallel to the floor. Or, you may find that your spine relaxes better and you're more comfortable with your knees bent and feet flat on the floor (see below).

2. Lengthen your spine and pull your shoulders down and away from your neck.

3. Close your eyes, breathe slowly and deeply from the abdomen, and imagine you're sinking into the floor with each breath. If you're new to relaxation techniques and your muscles are very tense, work slowly upwards from your toes and calves, getting each part of your body to relax.

4. Finish by looking downwards under your closed eyelids and feel the skin on your cheeks and forehead moving outwards and downwards towards the floor.

5. Open your eyes after fifteen minutes or so, and move on to first one side and then the other before you get up . . . very slowly.

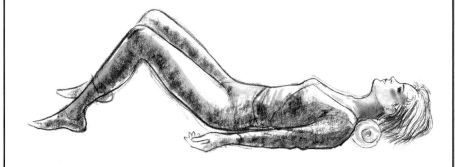

The forward curl

If you don't have time to do the yoga relaxation, try this: stand with bare feet hip-width apart. Slowly curl down, moving each vertebra gently as you bend forward, until your head is as close to your knees as you can comfortably reach. Lightly shake your head and neck to release any tension. Breathe in and out slowly and remain in this forward bend for thirty seconds to a minute, then tighten your stomach muscles and uncurl each vertebra very slowly until you are standing up straight once more.

Bach flower remedies

Tranquillisers, like sleeping pills, are not an effective long term solution. If you need some extra help to get you to unwind, try the instant tension reliever that is totally natural and non-addictive. A few drops of Bach Rescue Remedy relieves panic and all its side effects and makes you feel able to cope with anything. Rescue Remedy is made from essences of Cherry Plum, Clematis, Impatiens, Rock Rose and Star of Bethlehem. A few drops in water or on your tongue will make the world seem an easier place to live in.

MASSAGE

Massage stimulates the circulation, unlocks muscle tension and encourages relaxation. While it's important to pay a professional to give you a proper massage, it's very soothing to have a gentle-handed partner using oil and long, smooth strokes with the palms, always moving towards the heart. Tight shoulders (such a tension target) will release a little with squeezing and sliding movements using the pads of thumbs and fingers and moving from outer edge to neck. Don't leap up after a massage. In fact, it's best fitted in between a late night bath and bed.

Relieve headaches

Head massage relieves tension headaches and relaxes the face – you can do this one for yourself:

Use the pads of your fingertips and thumbs and start just above the ears making small circling movements, moving upwards to the crown.(Don't drag fingers over hair, just move the flesh of the scalp over the skull.) Work all over your head.

Finish by gently pressing across the base of the skull where it meets the neck. Start just behind the ears, press with your thumbs, move along a little, press again. Continue until the thumbs meet at mid-neck.

SLEEP

Hit the pillow for less than your usual sleeping hours or spend a few restless nights, and you'll face your waking hours puffy eyed and pale (and we won't mention your touchy temper, lack of concentration and general 'hang dog' look). But just how much sleep we need varies from person to person.

Most adults aim for around eight hours out of twenty-four, some function at full throttle on four and others need ten. Age influences our sleep requirements. A newborn baby may just eat, get cleaned up and sleep (if you're lucky), but a toddler can drive you to exhaustion for twelve hours a day! During the teenage years, that lively child will be almost impossible to prise from bed and those long hours of rest will be needed for a growing, changing body. Most of us demand shorter nights as we grow older, although the after-lunch, heavy eyelid syndrome usually develops into a series of catnaps with greater age and opportunity.

Sleep comes at several levels. After the first light doze, it gets deeper, progressing to the deepest level and rising again to the lighter dream phase. These dreamless deep and dream-filled lighter levels alternate throughout the night. During the deep sleep phase, your body recoups and restores itself. In the lighter, dreaming phase (and even if you don't remember your dreams you still dream) you work out your worries including things you've refused to face up to during your waking hours. Adequate, untroubled sleep is vital for physical and mental health.

Sleeping pills are not a long term answer to insomnia. Your body grows accustomed to them within weeks, and they can become addictive and leave you feeling low the next day. They can also have side effects, including skin rashes and blemishes. Even the occasional sleeping pill, taken if you're going through a stressful phase, will knock you out rather than bring the healthy and restorative highs and lows of natural sleep.

Try to woo sleep naturally. Wind down before bed, maybe using the yoga relaxation technique. Great sleep-inducers are: a good slice of exercise during the day, a contented mind, a soothing pursuit like listening to music, a warm bath, a firm, but comfortable bed, a loving bedfellow, and a hot drink.

Go for herbal tea, malted or chocolate drinks and avoid stimulating coffee or strong cups of tea. An occasional small alcoholic drink may help you to find sleep, but regularly knocking back many before bed will do the opposite.

Read a book at bedtime provided that it's not frightening, exciting or so good you can't bear to put it down.

If you really can't get to sleep, try to rest or read either a boring or very erudite book (both can make your mind switch off). By resting horizontally, you are getting many of the benefits of sleep. If you just can't settle, get up, tackle a task, and catch up on your lost slumbers the next night.

POSITIVE THINKING

Most of us have met the still-young eighty year-old who gives and gets so much from life, and the twenty year-old who's gone from childhood to immediate middle age with no joyful in-between stage.

Projecting a youthful image – whatever your chronological age – depends on vitality, a zest for living and an interest in other people and in yourself. Ask yourself if you're nice to know. Are you interesting, a pleasant companion, colleague, partner, mother, or lover? Look for the good things in your life and in other people. (This doesn't mean you have to be a pushover who takes all the flack from anyone in your life range who insists on taking a nasty and negative view of the world.) But, if you see the best in people, it will make your life less stressful. Giving and taking love and affection breeds contentment, and makes you look younger longer.

Having a wonderful time is a great energiser too. So, go on, enjoy yourself, do things you want to do and perhaps haven't dared to before. If you can't get out of something you hate doing, try to find its positive side – even if it's only a laugh. Laughter is a positive face lifter, whereas discontent drags you and your features down in every way.

THE BARE FACTS

It's surprisingly easy to forget about much of your body skin for large parts of the year if you live in a cold or cold-ish climate. Okay, *you* may be a regular swimmer, a strip-down keep-fitter, or have a job that involves being seen in public wearing very little, but for most of us as long as we're in reasonable shape and don't have a chronic skin problem, clothes can help us forget blotches, blemishes, minor sags and dried-up, grey looking body skin until we're suddenly faced with a bare-a-lot holiday or an evening do when a deep decolleté can easily announce your neglect of your skin to the rest of the world.

So, even if you're conserving energy or money by keeping the home fires low, make sure one room is warm enough for a regular strip down in front of a full-length mirror to give yourself a reminder that skin care should be a top-to-toe business carried out on a daily basis.

COLD WEATHER SKIN CARE

When the temperature drops:

- Get out of hibernation and into circulation! Wear layers of light, loose clothing that trap the warmth from your body between them. Whatever the weather, don't spend too much time in tight clothes – apart from encouraging circulation problems, varicose veins and thigh fat troubles (more on that subject later), they can abrade the skin, and encourage dryness and flaking.

- Wear clothes made from natural fibres which discourage and absorb perspiration better than man-made ones. Hairy knits can irritate your skin and may encourage you to scratch and disturb it – so wear a silk or cotton blouse or T-shirt under sweaters.

- Start your day with a few minutes of hectic exercising (see opposite).

- Never mind the weather! Give yourself a daily walk with arms swinging and head held high.

- Warming winter food doesn't have to wreck your healthy eating plans. Make pots of vegetable soup, eat rice, pasta and jacket potatoes with natural yoghurt and a tasty filling. Do keep up your daily fresh fruit and vegetable intake.

BEAUTY AND THE BATH

Follow these lines and discover the regenerative effects of 'taking the waters':

- Take a bath if you're tense, have been exercising or just feel ready for a good night's sleep, but don't overdo your soaking time – ten minutes is enough, more will dry out your skin. Showers are less taxing for your skin, so take one instead of a bath at least every other day – more if your skin is naturally dry or mature.

- Work on stimulating circulation and smoothing your skin by using a loofah, massage mitt, brush, exfoliating sponge or body scrub at least once a week. Avoiding the breasts, move towards the heart – up the arms, legs and trunk. Concentrate on the wrinkly bits, the elbows and knees and your back, which can be an oily area, often prone to spots. Monitor the process if you have a sensitive skin, to check that such treatments aren't too harsh for it.

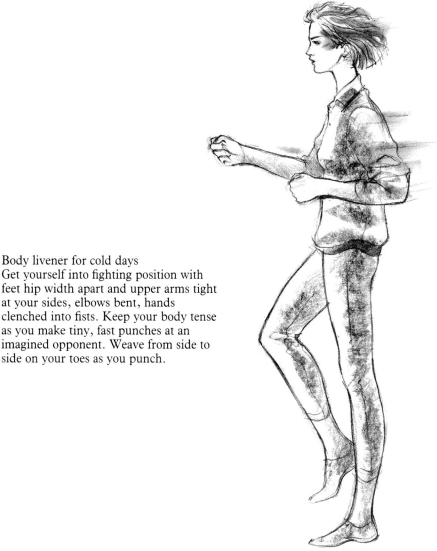

Body livener for cold days
Get yourself into fighting position with
feet hip width apart and upper arms tight
at your sides, elbows bent, hands
clenched into fists. Keep your body tense
as you make tiny, fast punches at an
imagined opponent. Weave from side to
side on your toes as you punch.

- Your bath water should be just comfortably warm. Over-hot water is a
  strain on the heart and the skin, and will encourage veins, dry skin, and
  the ageing process. Whether you bathe or shower, a cold water spray
  makes a healthy finish to the process and stimulates circulation.

- If you love to be accompanied in the bath by bubbles, gels or creams
  look for ones where the detergent is made from ingredients that are kind
  to the skin like coconut oil or cocoa butter.

89

- Many simple, inexpensive products can be used in the bath to improve the surface of your skin: a cup of cider vinegar will soothe dry, irritated skin; a cup of powdered milk will smooth and heal rough skin; a handful of cooking salt will alleviate minor skin problems; a cup of oatmeal or bran neatly controlled in a muslin bag and rubbed over the body is an age-old recipe for cleansing, whitening and soothing the skin.

- A handful of cooking salt mixed with a little oil (almond, sunflower or sesame are good, but any vegetable oil will do if you do not have these) rubbed over the body (avoiding the breasts) makes a first rate exfoliant. This is best done in the shower, so you can rinse the debris away afterwards.

- There is a large number of herbs that are kind to the skin and can be used in the bath. Here are a few that are easy to obtain. Either tie them in a muslin bag, so you don't leave the bath looking as though you've been dragged naked through the woods, or make an infusion with 2 or 3 tablespoons of the herb steeped in boiling water, left to cool, then strained and added to the bath. **Comfrey** softens and soothes the skin. **Camomile** calms mind and body. **Fennel** helps release impurities. **Lavender** and **Thyme** are antiseptic. **Marigold** is a well-known healer. **Mint** helps heal minor skin eruptions. **Rosemary** is a skin tonic.

- A few drops of essential oil (dealt with more fully in the section on aromatherapy) added to a warm bath provides a luxurious skin aid. Close all your doors and windows and inhale the aroma for five or ten minutes. Sandalwood, geranium, juniper, lavender, and chamomile are all excellent for the skin. If you have professional treatments, your aromatherapist may well suggest a mixture specifically made for you.

- Pat yourself dry after a bath if you want to unwind; rub yourself briskly if it's time to get moving. Always use a body moisturiser on dry areas, and use one from neck to toe if your skin is mature, or if you've been exposed to the sun.

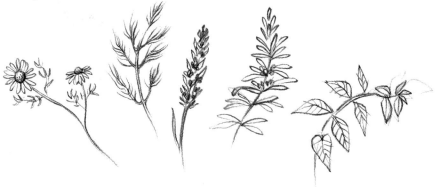

SPECIAL CARE FOR SPECIAL PLACES

Several skin factors affect the way you should treat your body. Backs, for example, are not in easy reach, and have far more sebaceous glands than the legs and arms so can easily become spot-ridden. Breasts are another area requiring special treatment as they have little more to hold them in shape than an envelope of supporting skin. Buttocks are highly pressurised (particularly the buttocks of those in sedentary jobs), but positioned so they can be easily forgotten. Hands and feet work hard every moment of the day, yet they're far from the central circulatory system, and tend to be last in line when the 'goodies' are scarce (which is why they feel the cold before the rest of you).

Jenny Travers, one of Clarins' leading skin care specialists, points out that the skin covering our bodies can be divided into two areas – the *dorsal* (tougher) and *ventral* (more delicate) types. Imagine you are on all fours. The part of your body then exposed to the sun or light – back, buttocks, and the outside of arms and legs is stronger and more resilient than the underparts – chest, stomach, and the insides of arms and legs. Always treat the more delicate skin with extra care, and protect it more highly from the sun.

THE BACK

The central area between the shoulders has a high sebum and perspiration output and due to its difficult placing can often miss out on thorough, regular, clean ups. Make sure you have the right tools for this job and work on it every time you bathe or shower. A long-handled back brush is best for the bath, a brush or massage back strap for the shower. If the area is very oily, powder lightly with talc. If the area is badly blemished, don't give it treatment with brushes or massage straps – follow medical advice.

Too great a body weight, lack of exercise and bad posture can give you ageing droops and lumps of flesh under shoulder blades (as well as many other problems). Keep your weight as near ideal as possible and take your exercise regularly. Stand and sit with the spine stretched upwards, the head lifted away from the body, shoulders gently back and down so they move inwards towards the spine. Due to bad posture, most people over the age of twelve or so have some misalignment of the spine which affects every part of the body. One way to combat this is to follow a course in the Alexander Technique which would vastly improve health, posture, and looks and obviate much back pain and discomfort (see page 172 for the address of the Society of Teachers of the Alexander Technique).

Badly fitting bras affect the look of your back and shoulders. A strap which is too tight will encourage bulges above and below, a bra that relies on straps rather than shaping to hold you in place can cut furrows into your shoulders. For the sake of your back and bust try to get bras fitted by a trained expert.

THE BREASTS

Whether you're large busted or built on the lines of a boy, your breasts rely for support on a tenuous connection with the underlying chest muscles, ligaments and the envelope of covering skin that goes from under your breasts up to the jaw line.

Swimming is the best possible bust conditioner, bringing exercise without the downward pull of gravity. If you can plough up and down a pool for twenty minutes three or four times a week you will, barring ill-health, keep breasts in good shape for life.

It is important always to wear a flexible but supporting bra when you exercise on dry land or you'll be swinging the weight of your breasts and stretching the supporting ligaments and skin. It is a very good idea to add a morning stint of bust-enhancing exercise to any regular routine. Opposite is one of the simplest and best which also exercises upper arm muscles.

Keep your weight as constant as possible – weight variations can lead to inflation, deflation and subsequent stretch marks on the delicate skin of the breasts. During pregnancy and breast feeding, monitor your bust size and buy bras which will fit well and support adequately. Your breasts may increase in size before menstruation. Be aware of this as you may need a larger bra for this time.

Take expert advice when dealing with your bust support. Buy bras from shops with expert fitters (or at the very least where you'll get good advice). When you lift you arms up, your bra band should stay in place, no part should press into your flesh, and cups should be comfortably filled, not straining or half empty. Padded bras can encourage excessive perspiration which adversely affects the skin. A restrictive bra prevents efficient circulation in the area, and a bra which is too large or elderly won't support breasts.

Going bra-less from time to time is fine if you are reasonably young and not over-endowed. Large and older breasts need support whenever you're standing up to prevent their weight from accelerating their fall. Going bra-less on the beach when you're running around or playing games is not a

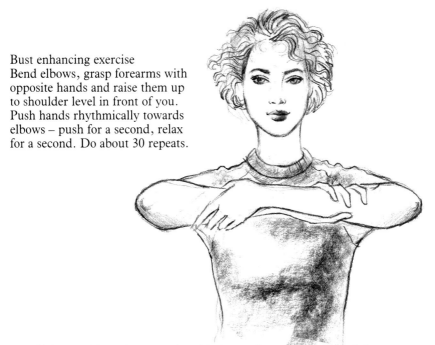

Bust enhancing exercise
Bend elbows, grasp forearms with
opposite hands and raise them up
to shoulder level in front of you.
Push hands rhythmically towards
elbows – push for a second, relax
for a second. Do about 30 repeats.

good idea and bare breasts should always be well protected from exposure to the sun.

Many beauty salons in Britain now give bust treatments to help firm and tone the supporting skin. Apart from the treatment you will learn a lot about your bust, how to look after it at home, and how to properly apply moisturisers and toning products. Never lie in the bath with breasts submerged – you'll dry out and ruin the condition of the skin. After bathing or showering, dry breasts gently and very thoroughly, paying particular attention underneath if they are heavy and low on your ribcage, using a soft towel working clockwise around the circumference and upwards towards the throat. Apply moisturiser or bust toning lotion with the same upward movement. Just being aware of your breasts as you work on them could well help improve their condition.

If you're feeling down or depressed, your bust can reflect those feelings. Many body therapists have noticed how breasts collapse, and the covering skin becomes cold and flabby, when a woman is ill or unhappy. When you're feeling well again and loved and contented your breasts will regain their bouncy quality and lively skin.

A sprinkling of hair around the nipples of a woman's breasts is quite normal. These can be cut carefully or removed by electrolysis but *never* pluck hairs in this area. You risk distorting the follicle and encouraging ingrowing hairs in this delicate skin.

THE BUTTOCKS

Buttocks suffer from their place on the body map. We're usually unhappy about sagging bottoms, but it's a vague feeling most of the time and the buttocks are easy enough to forget. Yet this is an important area both aesthetically – bulges and droops look bad with or without a covering of cloth – and physically, as the bottom is vital in its interaction between back and thighs. It's a rewarding spot to work on too, as it has strong skin and muscles that respond quickly to treatment.

Don't miss out on the buttock area when you're exfoliating your body – get to work with a massage mitt every time you bath or shower to improve local circulation, texture and tone. Be lavish with moisturiser, as contact between hard surfaces, clothes and flesh when you're sitting bring constant friction that can upset the skin's surface. Follow the anti-cellulite advice to keep dimpling at bay and try some of these tightening exercises for thighs and buttocks:

Standing slim
Practise tucking the buttocks under when you stand – sticking them out makes them look larger and puts a strain on your back. Stand sideways on to a mirror and move your pelvis back and forward like a belly dancer. When the lower part is tilted forwards, you'll see how much slimmer your behind and stomach look.

Big squeeze
Go for the 'big squeeze'. Several times a day, no matter whether you're sitting or standing, rhythmically tense and release your buttock muscles.

Shaping up
Get down on your hands and knees a couple of times a day for some moves that will help to shape up hips and thighs as well as buttocks:

1. Kneel on all fours with arms in a straight line under shoulders, knees under hips. Keep your buttocks level and spine in a straight line from head to coccyx as you straighten out one leg behind you, flexing the foot so that your toes point towards the floor (see opposite). Lift the straight leg eight times without lifting or tilting the hip. Replace knee on the floor and do the straight leg lifts with the other leg. Repeat the eight lifts five times each side.

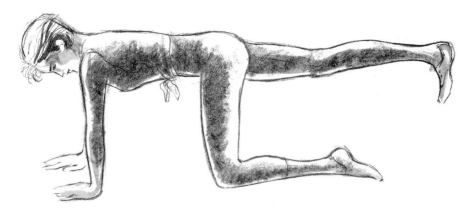

Shaping up exercise 1

2. Remain kneeling in the same way for the following exercise known as 'Rover's Revenge' (you'll see how it gets its name when you do it) – it is great for tightening the inner thighs and buttocks: Lift one bent leg sideways as far as possible, and return it to the kneeling leg, but don't rest it on the floor. Repeat the lift swiftly sixteen times. Do 3 × 16 lifts with each leg.

Inner thighs

For tough measures on inner thighs and buttocks, try this one: sit on the floor with legs outstretched, ankles either side of chair legs. Now try to pull the ankles together. Alternatively, you can do this one standing up with feet either side of a large book – a telephone directory works well. Again, work your legs as though you are trying to pull the ankles together.

THE STOMACH

The abdominal area is packed with a criss cross network of muscles that are willing to work with the slightest encouragement. Here are some exercises to develop and strengthen them:

Looking slim

Stand with the lower pelvis tucked under as you're doing for buttocks and you'll automatically pull in your stomach area. Sit up in your chair with a straight spine, stomach held in. Slouching makes you look half a stone heavier and muscles go to pot.

Curl-ups

There's nothing like curl-ups, properly done, to beat stomach bulge. Lie on the floor with knees bent, feet flat on the floor, and hands at your sides. Make sure your back is flat on the floor, with no gaps under the waist area. Breathe in and as you breathe out, lift your head, shoulders and upper back from the floor, curving your spine and reaching towards your knees with straight arms. Hold for a second or two and breathe in as you lie back. Repeat the movement several times.

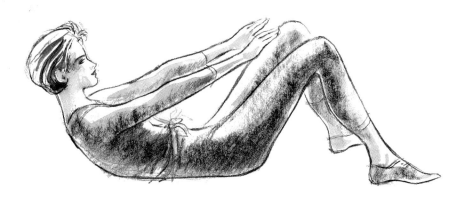

If your muscles are already strong, or as they strengthen, try this more advanced version. Lift head, shoulders and upper back as before, and from that raised position slowly move an inch back and an inch forward. Try to do thirty of these backward and forward moves before you curl back to the floor.

Waist bends

Exercise the muscles of your waist with side bends. Stand with feet hip width apart. Tighten your buttocks so your hips remain still during side bends. (They should not thrust out on the opposite side to your down bend.) Hold your hands above your head with arms straight. As you bend, the arms move over to assist the bend. Repeat the side bends about twenty times, straightening arms and spine between each bend.

During pregnancy, the skin of the abdominal area takes considerable strain. Generally, darker, tougher skins expand more easily than pale, delicate ones and whether you are left with stretch marks is greatly governed by hormones, your size during pregnancy and your skin type. But give the upper layers as much moisturising help as possible by gently

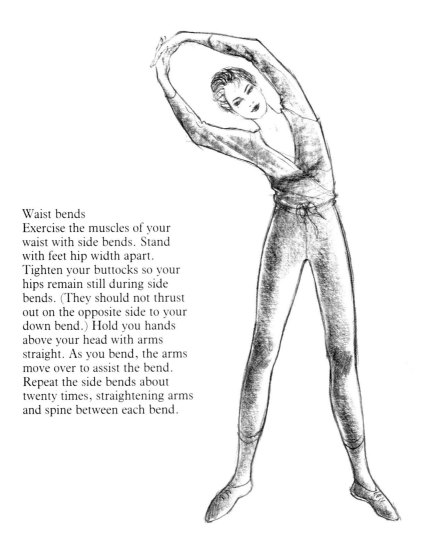

Waist bends
Exercise the muscles of your
waist with side bends. Stand
with feet hip width apart.
Tighten your buttocks so your
hips remain still during side
bends. (They should not thrust
out on the opposite side to your
down bend.) Hold you hands
above your head with arms
straight. As you bend, the arms
move over to assist the bend.
Repeat the side bends about
twenty times, straightening arms
and spine between each bend.

massaging with vegetable oils a couple of times a day during the expansion
time. Start exercises after the birth as soon as your doctor says you may.

Many women and men have a tendency to put on localised weight
around the abdomen, particularly as they reach middle age, even if they
are not overweight elsewhere. Nutritionist Celia Wright terms this allergic
oedema – your body does not happily accept one or more of the foods you
are eating. Try the Refresher Course (see page 66) and see localised fat
melt away (at least it did for me and several other testers). As you go back to
a normal diet, introduce food types one at a time, so you can tell which
foods disagree with your body.

THE FEET

Even unenthusiastic walkers clock up something like 70,000 miles in an average lifespan and those flexible, hard-working feet take your weight every moment you're on them. Look after your feet and legs, and the whole of you will stay looking young and lively.

Shoes should be at least a quarter of an inch longer than the foot with room for the toes to spread comfortably. They should fit snugly at the heel and instep. Your feet pour out a cup a water a day – so give shoes a twenty-four hour airing between wears. Change tights, socks, and stockings at least once a day. Use special foot powder before putting on footwear, as talc is too fine to be efficient and absorbent. Keep high heels for occasional wear, as they interfere with the natural balance of your feet and body. Sling-backs and mules don't hold your heel in place properly, and frequent wearings will lead to callouses on the under heel area.

Corns and callouses are caused by shoes which press and interfere with circulation. Buy footwear late in the day, not early when feet are at their thinnest and best. Refer corns and hard skin problems to a good chiropodist, never try to hack at them yourself. Do give yourself a regular pedicure, cutting toe nails straight across. Follow these tips for healthy feet!

- Go barefoot whenever it is possible, and safe.

- If you press hardest on the ball or heel of your foot you will naturally develop callouses where the pressure is greatest. Yoga lessons are a great way to learn how to utilise the entire foot for correct balance. This will strengthen ankles and insteps too.

- Take the pressure off your feet and legs by lying down with your feet high above your head for ten minutes. This is also a great boost for your kidneys and eliminatory system. Do this as a refresher during the day if possible. Always try to put your feet up for ten minutes immediately before you pop between the sheets at night, particularly if you're inclined to varicose veins.

- Feet and legs are low in sebaceous glands. A massage with a rich body lotion will take away tiredness and minor aches and make up for the natural oil deficiencies in this area. Massage from base to tip of each toe, across the top of the feet and upwards from ankles to knees.

THE HANDS

Run a home, a family, do almost any job, play games and go outdoors in all weather and your hands are first in line for hard times. Like feet, they are out on a limb, last in line for sustenance from the central circulatory system, and they're far from rich in sebaceous glands and natural oil supply. They need constant care and protection or they can signal your age (and add years to it) before any other part of you. Here are some ways to help you keep your hands smooth and looking good:

- Wear gloves whenever possible when you're outdoors. In summer, treat your hands to high protection sunscreens.

- Avoid hand contact with harsh chemicals, dirt and long soaking sessions in water. Wear protective gloves whenever you're doing dirty or wet work indoors or out. When you're wearing rubber gloves, choose ones with a cotton lining to soak up skin-spoiling perspiration.

- Lash on moisturiser and hand cream whenever you think of it – hands can't have enough. When you manicure, finish with a massage movement and hand cream – up each finger and thumb from base to tip and across tops of hands from centre to sides.

- Perk up work-worn, grimy hands with a teaspoon of castor sugar and a little vegetable oil massaged in with firm strokes and rubbed around the fingers with the thumb and forefinger of your opposite hand. Rinse off with warm water and reach for your favourite hand cream. Dried-out, flaking nails will benefit from a ten minute soak in warm olive oil.

- Keep fingers flexible, and release tension with some hand exercises. Get a squash ball or a child's rubber ball that's slightly smaller than a tennis ball and squeeze it while you're doing nothing more active than sitting watching TV. Then bend your knuckles and press each finger gently with the thumb and forefinger of the other hand. Do a few finger press ups by laying your hand flat on a solid surface with fingers spread, then lifting the palm off the surface, so that the back of the hand is at right angles to the fingers.

- Let your hands help you to tranquillity using this exercise (see the illustration on the next page). Grip the fleshy part between the thumb and forefinger of one hand with the thumb and forefinger of the other. Press into the fleshy area with your thumb and make tiny circles for a count of ten seconds, then release for three seconds. Repeat three times on each hand. You'll feel much calmer afterwards and it's just the thing to stop your stomach churning at moments of high anxiety.

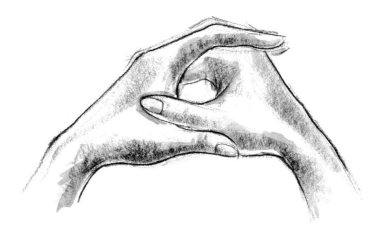

Tranquillity exercise
Pinch the fleshy area between the thumb and forefinger of one hand with the
thumb and forefinger of the other hand and make tiny circular movements with the
thumb for ten seconds. Then release. Repeat three times on each hand.

FIGHT CELLULITE

Read a dozen articles on the subject of cellulite and each one seems to give a
different explanation – including total denial that such a condition exists.
But, look around any beach and, unless most of the females are young,
sleek and super-fit, you'll see some degree of puckered, quilted flesh on
their thighs and whatever part of their buttocks that is visible. Men can be
ancient, unfit and overweight and yet most of them miss out on the problem flesh.

It is a fact that nearly all females have a high fat cell content in the area of
their thighs and pelvis. At puberty, the cells increase in volume and the
skin thickens, but – just as some women have large breasts, others small –
some have controllable fat on the thighs, while others have a greater cellulite potential. With age, hormone changes, neglect and abuse, a biological
go-slow starts the build up. Fat and fluid retention inhibit circulation,
there's localised difficulty with taking up oxygen and getting rid of waste
products, and the connective tissue around the fatty deposits loses flexi-
bility. Nothing works well or holds together smoothly. Eventually the area
resembles its graphic French description, *peau d'orange* or orange peel. It
gets quilted, puckered, dimpled and ugly to look at. The tendency to
develop cellulite is inherited, and any hormone upheavels such as pregnancy, the Pill and menopause can compound the condition, as can a
sedentary lifestyle, poor elimination, bad eating habits, alcohol, stress and
lack of exercise. Prevention and control are far better than any attempts at

cure when it's firmly in place and it's much easier to check its development when you're young. But, while cellulite is always hard to move, it can be helped on its way if you're willing to work regularly at it.

How to fight cellulite

- **Get off your butt.** Women athletes very rarely suffer from cellulite, so take regular exercise which replaces fat with muscle, and improves circulation, elimination and your breathing techniques. The best anti-cellulite exercises are swimming (the movement of legs through water gives them a gentle massage too), fast walking, particularly hill walks, tightening exercise such as cycling – either the real thing, a stationary exercise bike or just doing a daily session of a hundred pedalling movements when you're lying on your back. Long sessions of sitting and standing encourage the problem, so if these are a large part of your daily round, make a particular point of getting some movement into your life. Always sit well back in a hard chair. Constantly perching on the edge encourages a permanent pressure bulge at the back of the thigh.

- **Stick to a healthy food intake** that includes a high percentage of fresh, uncooked foods daily, and avoid tinned, processed, refined, smoked and pickled foods. Cut down (or preferably out) alcohol, coffee, strong tea and cigarettes. Aromatherapist Eve Taylor who has worked on bodies all over the world, has found that heavy thighs and/or cellulite problems seem to respond to foods low in animal fats. Try cutting out butter, high fat cheeses and fatty meats. Substitute fish, poultry, vege-table fat and lots of raw fruit and vegetables.

- **Drink plenty of the right liquids** – fresh fruit and vegetable juices, herb teas, and mineral water. Try a diuretic drink made from liquidising a handful of fresh parsley, a few lettuce leaves and a stick of celery. Top it up with mineral water.

- **Relaxation** and a positive lifestyle can help. Research suggests that stress, anxiety, depression and poor sleeping habits are conducive to the development of cellulite.

- **Massage** helps move the mass, but don't expect overnight miracles. Best and most luxurious is aromatherapy which restores balance to the whole body, and improves elimination and circulation. There are many products sold specifically for home treatment. Most contain ivy, horse chestnut or seaweed extracts – all reputedly enemies of cellulite – and are designed to be used with massage movements. If you are using these products without a massage glove or applicator, perfect your own techniques. First use gentle upward strokes from knee to thigh for a couple of minutes, then gently clench your hands and work upwards from the knee massaging with the middle knuckles and small, circular movements as your hands travel upwards to the tops of your thighs.

- **Hydrotherapy**   If you have a high pressure shower you can have a little hydrotherapy at home. Direct the jet up the thighs and across the pelvic area.

- **Clothing**   Make sure clothes are comfortable and not constricting, particularly around the thighs, buttocks and waistband.

- **Liposuction** or fat aspiration permanently removes a certain number of fat cells and is now an established, if expensive and fairly extreme method of reducing and re-shaping heavy thighs. Liposuction is not an answer to advanced cellulite and skin elasticity has to be good for complete success.

Have you got cellulite?

If you slide the palm of your hand up the thigh with a lifting movement and it smooths out, you don't have cellulite, just out-of-condition thighs. But, the treatment is the same and, providing skin elasticity is reasonable, it's easier to improve than the real thing.

You can test your cellulite possibilities even if it's not obvious. Lay both your hands flat on one thigh about three inches apart with fingers pointing towards the knee. Push the hands towards one another and early cellulite will show up on the squeezed piece of flesh.

CHAPTER FIVE

YOUR SKIN AND THE SUN

Happily the sixties and seventies fashion for madly overdone tans has given way to gentler shades of gold. But, give most of us a chance to take time off in the sun and we'll still cast aside all caution and words of warning with our clothes. Unfortunately there are, as yet, no government health warnings about the long-term harm ultra violet rays can do to the skin and we still equate browning our bodies with health and glamour. We persist in *cultivating* a tan when we should look upon it as a sideline to having a super time outdoors.

Dr John Hawk, Head of the Photobiology Department at St Thomas' Hospital in London, says, 'A sun tan has no health benefits other than psychological. Ultra violet rays cause temporary sunburn damage to the outer, self-replacing layers of the skin, and permanent, progressive damage to the basal layer and dermis. They are a major factor in premature ageing, and other cosmetic and important skin problems. But the outdoor life is healthy, and recreation in sunlight enjoyable. By all means carry on swimming, sailing, water skiing, wind surfing, and playing games on the beach. But do protect your skin. People won't and can't stay out of the sun, but they can minimise the potential harm it can do to skin. Try to stay indoors when the sun is high in the sky as in the middle part of the day, particularly when you visit sub-tropical climates. Be very careful when you first expose your body to the sun after the winter, but your skin can become naturally between 10 and 40 times better protected at the end of a holiday. Wear a high SPF sunscreen on all exposed areas and repeat the application every hour or so when you're outdoors and always after swimming and exercise.'

DON'T BE HALF BAKED

The sun bombards the earth with ultra violet rays – UVC, UVA and UVB. UVC is lethal to cells, but does not get through the earth's atmosphere. UVA tans well, burns only a little, but penetrates the skin deeply, and tends to cause long-term damage such as wrinkling and may exacerbate the cancer threat of UVB rays. UVB tans, burns easily, but penetrates less deeply. UVA rays are very constant during the day, UVB are more intense in the middle of the day when the sun is high in the sky.

Given no escalating problems with the ozone layer, the earth's atmosphere works as our first 'sunscreen', filtering UVB rays more effectively when the sun is low in the sky when they have further to travel through the atmosphere. Peak peril time is the three hours or so around noon and, of course, the nearer the equator you get, the greater the UVB intensity – Florida will fry you more thoroughly than Frinton for a larger part of the middle of the day.

Don't let clouds lull you into a false sense of security – you can easily get burned while wingeing about the weather on a dull and chilly day in summer. UVB is intensified by reflection from water, snow, sand and white surfaces, so you're doing nothing for your skin if you ski with an unprotected face or put up a big beach brolly and decide to eat a picnic lunch by the sea. Swimming affords no protection either – the burning rays penetrate underwater, and bits of you will be flashing around above sea level anyway.

If you have to be out in a hot midday sun – sightseeing or walking – cover up with loose, cotton clothes or a sarong bought or made from a 2–3m length of wide, fine cotton (no man-made fibres if you want comfort in the heat). Pop on a wide-brimmed hat and sunglasses and don't forget to wear a sunscreen on any exposed bits of you. Take some sunscreen with you for topping up your protection level.

NATURAL DEFENCES

While we're all vulnerable under the sun, some skins are more vulnerable than others. Your hair colouring does not necessarily indicate how your skin will react to sunlight. For example you may be blonde and yet not burn easily or brunette with a sun-shy skin. So, decide your type by the way your skin reacts to sunlight. These are the basic categories:

Type	Classification	Reaction	Examples
1	Sensitive	burns easily, never tans	red hair, freckled
2	Sensitive	burns easily, tans a little	fair, blue eyed
3	Normal	burns moderately, tans slowly	brown hair and eyes
4	Normal	can burn, tans well	Mediterranean
5	Non-sensitive	rarely burns, tans deeply	Middle Eastern Asian
6	Non-sensitive	never burns, deeply pigmented	Afro-Caribbean

It's fairly certain that types 1 and 2 will do some damage to their skins after half an hour's midday sunning without protection, even in Britain. But even easy tanners can get an unexpected reaction to hot sun after months of being muffled in winter wear. There are many shades of Asian and black skins of course but the average black skin has 10–15 times more natural protection than the average white one.

Skin categories are one thing, skin condition is another. Always consider your skin, the time, the place and your degree of acclimatisation. Coming to terms with the sun, and being able to enjoy it with the minimum short and long term damage is always a matter of common sense, personal monitoring and under rather than overdoing exposure time.

SUN IN YOUR EYES

Good, tinted lenses protect your eyes from harmful rays and cut out glare from reflecting surfaces such as snow, sand, water, pavements, and white-washed buildings. Excessive eye exposure to ultra violet rays can give you headaches, nausea, sore, irritated eyes and even more serious problems. Tinted lenses can help to prevent you from squinting in the sunshine – which encourages wrinkles to form.

Fair-skinned people are sometimes the owners of sun-sensitive eyes. While your skin will soon tell you if it's sun-shy, your eyes may not do so for many years, and much damage may have been done by the time you realise this On the other hand, most eyes can make it safely through the average British summer uncovered, and constantly wearing tinted lenses can make eyes ultra-sensitive to light.

It's important to go to an optician for even non-prescription lenses, so you get expert advice on the degree of sun-sensitivity of your eyes and the best type(s) of tinted lenses for your eyes, the parts of the world where you'll be wearing them and their impact resistance qualities.

If you own any sunglasses that were purchased without expert advice, test the lenses this way. Hold the frame at arm's length and, looking through one lens at a time, focus on a slim vertical object such as a lamp-post or window edge. Rotate the lens and the vertical object should remain still. If it seems to move or alter shape, the lens is distorted and will do nothing for your vision.

EASY DOES IT

What happens when the sun's rays hit our pasty, newly uncovered bodies? Ouch, says the skin and proceeds to build up a defence mechanism by getting the pigment cells to increase production of melanin which is taken up to the surface where it darkens the skin's natural tone. At the same time, the outermost horny layer of the epidermis thickens to provide a stronger physical barrier. This is a fairly slow and progressive process, so give it a week or two.

Apart from the more immediate and obvious effects of over exposure, such as singed skin, the sun's rays start to degrade the lower reaches. Unprotected sun exposure at twenty years old may not show up for fifteen years or so, but suddenly the results are there – uneven brown blotches, less elasticity, and wrinkles that have arrived years before they should. Even worse, constant unprotected sunning can cause many nasty skin problems, including cancer.

While the sun is not a major source of skin problems in temperate Britain, cheaper travel and more leisure time has now made it so for travellers abroad. Dermatologists find that indoor workers who make a quick dash to the Mediterranean and peel off for long periods in the sun are literally risking their skins. Babies and young children are another high risk area. It's practically impossible to keep them in the shade once they're moving of their own volition and young skins have no history of facing up to sun, and their cells are growing and dividing, and are more susceptible to serious problems from ultra violet exposure.

These relatively new opportunities to bare ourselves in parts of the world where the sun shines more fiercely than here, have been balanced slightly by the enormous developments in sunscreens that provide physical and/or chemical filters that reflect or absorb UV light and help to increase our skin's protection against the sun's rays.

Sunscreen factors

Most suntan preparations use a system of numbers which denote their Sun Protection Factor (SPF). If you'd normally run in from the sun after 15 minutes, a product numbered 6 will increase that time to about 90 minutes (15 mins × 6); one numbered 8 to about two hours (15 mins × 8). The factor system has run wild recently with SPFs of 50 or more now appearing in the States. So simplification is the latest move with manufacturers being recommended to add descriptions like Intensive, High, Medium and Low Protection. Do check that your sunscreen also offers a high degree of UVA protection. Look for three (superior) or four stars (maximum) cover whatever the SPF rating (which refers only to the degree of protection against UVB). Dermatologists suggest that SPF 12–15 is as high as you're likely to need unless you're allergic to the sun. After all you *will* be re-applying after an hour, not expecting it to last for ten.

Tender parts

Whether you're dealing with words or numbers, go for more protection than you think you need, particularly on vulnerable parts of the body such as your neck, shoulders, tops of feet, breasts and nipples (if you're going topless), breastbone and your face which spends its life dealing with UV rays. It's wise to use a foundation or moisturiser all year round – even in temperate Britain – that contains UV filters.

Men with short hair cuts should protect the tips of their ears, and those not thickly thatched should wear a sun hat or cover any bald part with a high protection sunscreen. Children spend hours digging in the sand, so take extra care with backs, shoulders and cheeks that can catch the rays.

Sunscreens don't greatly prevent your skin from changing to a darker shade. They do increase protection and the time you can spend in the sun without burning and badly damaging your skin.

Be prepared

Unless you know your holiday area and what you can buy there, take your sun care products with you in case you find yourself somewhere where good ones that cope with both UVA and UVB rays are difficult or impossible to find. Choose from creams, milks, lotions, blocks or gels and go for waterproof lotion if you're off to a beach and sea holiday or if you perspire quite heavily – it's very much a question of preference and using the appropriate screening factors. Oils tend to have low sun protection factors, smack a little of 'Who's frying to-day?' and are not suitable for sensitive skins. At least one manufacturer has thought of the games people play and has come up with a waterproof, water-based sunscreen to stop you skidding off surfboards or rackets and clubs slipping out of your hand. Its oil-free formula makes it useful for hairy bodied males and heads where the hair is thinning. When you come in from the sun, use a special after-sun shower product and lash on lots of after-sun lotion to combat the drying effects of the sun.

If a tan is what you really want, pre-tan activators or accelerators may attract you. Tests suggest they don't do much more than add a little moisture. If you hate showing off a white body try fake tans. Fake tans work by a chemical process that changes the colour of the outer-most layers of the skin. They wear off as the outer skin is shed. Most of them look fairly realistic these days, so by all means use them if you want to look less of an outsider on the beach.

Sunbeds work rather like the UV rays of the sun. If you use them you will be exposing yourself to all the hazards connected with UV rays without having the fresh air and fun of being in the sun. They don't thicken the horny layer of the epidermis, so they don't put you too many points ahead with protection before you start a holiday. Save your money for a relaxing, fresh air break from routine rather than a sunbed.

If you have got burnt . . .

It takes about 6 to 8 hours for your body to let you know how much it hated you leaving it so long in the sun. Scorched, sore skin that feels as though it has been on a nutmeg grater is your pay-off. And if you've gone the far side of sun sense it can give you pain, blisters, puffiness, headaches and nausea. Stay out of the sun completely until you and your skin are better. Shower with tepid water, drink plenty of liquids and lash on moisturiser or after-sun lotion. If you feel poorly after 24 hours indoors, take yourself off to a doctor.

SKIN ALLERGIES AND THE SUN

Holiday happiness can be hampered by a nasty, itchy rash called polymorphic light eruption, often more easily although wrongly called prickly heat or heat rash. It is an allergic reaction, triggered by UV radiation, to internal substances that would normally cause us little or no trouble. Citrus fruits, artificial sweeteners, non-alcoholic drinks and caffeine (in tea, coffee, cola) can also cause problems. You could also have an adverse reaction if you're on certain drugs including some sedatives, antibiotics and contraceptive pills. If you're having any medical treatment or taking any drugs, it's wise to have a word with your GP before you spend too much time in the sun.

Certain ingredients in perfumes don't mix well with the sun, so keep perfume and perfumed products for after dark, and never spend time in the sun after aromatherapy or you could end up with blotchy stains on the skin that persist for years.

THE GOOD NEWS

If you're feeling that sun-seeking is fraught with so many dangers that you'd be better off taking your holiday in a darkened room, here's some brighter news. Scientists suggest that sunlight increases the body's production of endorphins (these are the happy hormones), and reduces production of adrenalin, the stress hormone. There's also scientific credibility for that miserable feeling one gets during the dark January and February days in a British winter. It's called the SAD syndrome or Seasonal Affective Disorder. When exposed to bright light, sufferers improve very quickly.

A small exposure to the sun (it's estimated that something like fifteen minutes every other day in British-strength summer sunlight) supplies our bodies' requirements of vitamin D – which has a prime role in bone health. (On the other hand, a typical Western diet is reckoned to supply all our needs on that score even if we don't get the sunshine.) And, of course, sunlight is not all bad news for some skins. People who suffer from acne, psoriasis and eczema often find an improvement in their condition during the summer months. So, don't stay away from the sun, but remember that a little goes a very long way.

SUN, SNOW AND SKIING

Protection of exposed areas when skiing at high altitudes is even more essential than when you're playing in the sun during the summer. Your face takes the brunt of exposure, so protect this vulnerable area with a high SPF product specially formulated for high altitudes. Due to the thinner atmosphere, ultra-violet radiation will be intensified, so use a higher SPF than you do in the summer, and one that's made for the job.

High altitude protectors are specially formulated with a high oil, low water content. Low temperatures become much lower due to the wind chill factor when you're skiing at speed down a mountain – a high water content in products could freeze on your face. Also, water particles can increase the intensity of UV rays, so when it's snowing or foggy you're more at risk. Snow bounces the rays around too. Protect *under* your chin, nose and ears as well as over these areas. Be extra careful with lip protection and add plenty of rich moisturiser to your après-ski preparations.

The ten-point guide to safer summer sun

1. Take it slowly. Never go for the burn.

2. Make your sun time before 11 am and after 3 pm (GMT) especially in hot countries.

3. Use a High Protection sunscreen for initial exposure to the sun. You can reduce it slightly if you wish after a week.

4. Apply sunscreen just before you go in the sun, and re-apply every hour, after swimming, water sport or perspiring.

5. If you will be out at hot times sightseeing or on the water, wear cover up cotton clothes, high SPF sunscreens, a hat and sunglasses.

6. Drink plenty of bottled water when it's hot, and go easy on alcohol, tea, coffee, carbonated and citrus drinks.

7. Avoid wearing perfume and perfumed products.

8. Have a tepid shower, and lash on moisturiser when you come in from the sun.

9. Sun singed? Stay indoors for a couple of days. Get medical attention if you're feeling ill.

10. If you are taking any medically prescribed drugs, check with your doctor before you take on the sun.

CHAPTER SIX

*B*EAUTY TREATMENTS FOR SKIN AND BODY

*D*IY BEAUTY

Few people have the time or inclination to cook up their own face and body creams these days. But, if you're feeling frugal, and want a bit of fun, your kitchen holds plenty of products that will help soothe, smooth and beautify your skin without eating into precious time or more than a few pennies of the housekeeping budget.

Lemons
Lemons are rich in vitamin C, and also contain some of the Bs and E. They're natural bacteria fighters which is why diluted lemon plus honey is a help when you have a cold or 'flu symptoms. Used externally, they have astringent and mild bleaching properties. Stained and grubby hands, and off-colour cuticles and nail tips come clean if you rub them with a squeezed half of lemon. This will also remove smells on your hands if you've been peeling prawns, preparing fish or chopping onions and garlic. Always wash your hands in cold water first – as rinsing them in hot water will drive the smell in and your hands will waft unpleasing reminders of food preparation long after the meal is eaten and digested.

It's easy enough to dismiss much vaunted old remedies, but nothing rejuvenates long-neglected, hoary elbows as successfully as leaning them in squeezed-out lemon halves that contain a little cooking oil. Read a book for fifteen minutes or so while you take the treatment. Rub in some hand or body lotion when the lemon leaning session has finished.

A tiny drop of lemon juice can be used as antiseptic healer on the odd spot or two (test this very gently if you have a sensitive skin) and a few drops of lemon juice added to rosewater makes an antiseptic astringent for oily skin. Only add it to the rosewater you're going to use immediately, not to the bottle.

Lemon is great for you from top to toe. Tired feet revive when a squeezed half of lemon is rubbed over them and lemon peel rubbed over the teeth helps to remove stains caused by drinking tea, coffee and red wine. A sage leaf rubbed over teeth will help them to shine too, and a strawberry will gently clean them up and leave your mouth feeling fresh. (Follow your usual dental routine as well. They're an additional cleanser, not a substitute.)

Fresh fruit

Fresh fruit can be used as face packs for all types of skin. Strawberries, tomatoes, and apples soften and whiten the skin and gently control oiliness. Peaches, apricots and melon will soothe and moisturise. Grapes and pears have a cleansing effect. All citrus fruits are toning, astringent and antiseptic, but need to be used in diluted doses unless your skin is strong and oily. Slice or pulp the fruits and lay them over your freshly cleansed face for 15 minutes or so while you lie back with your feet up. (It's a good idea to put plastic over the pillow or cushion, so you don't scatter it with falling pieces of fruit.) When your time is up, remove the fruit, rinse with tepid water and apply moisturiser.

A strawberry milk shake makes a brightening cleanser for skins that are sallow or suffering from a fading suntan. Whisk up 2 oz of strawberries with half a pint of milk. Strain the mixture and wipe over your face with cotton wool. You can drink up the leftovers.

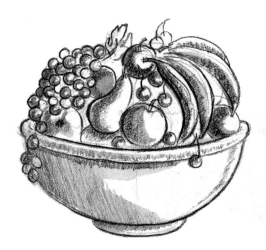

Eggs

Eggs are a prime source of protein, and also contain vitamins A, the B group, and E and D plus many minerals. Cosmetically, the white tones and refines the skin, whilst the contents of the yolk are compatible with the hair and skin and have a gently moisturising action.

For oily skins, whisk up the white and coat the face with it, leaving the eye area clear. When the white is dry, paint on the lightly beaten yolk. Relax for ten minutes. Remove with tepid water. For dry and delicate skins, use the yolk only, beaten up with a teaspoonful of glycerine and a little double cream. Again remove with tepid water after 10 minutes.

Pure honey

Honey is easily digested, and is an instant energy giver. Provided you know and trust your egg source, one of the quickest and most sustaining meals (and it tastes okay) is a raw egg beaten up with half a pint of milk and a teaspoonful or two of honey.

Used externally, runny honey makes a good moisturising agent. For dry and dehydrated skin beat up 3 dessertspoonfuls of cream with one of honey. Rinse off after 15 minutes.

For the tastiest mask that suits most skins, mix 2 teaspoonfuls of honey with 2 tablespoonfuls of natural yoghurt – you can make an extra large quantity and eat what's left. After the usual 10 to 15 minutes, remove with cotton wool and warm water.

Avocados

Dip into an avocado for more face masks. If your skin is dry, mash the flesh with a teaspoon of honey; if it's oily add the same amount of lemon juice instead. Rinse the mask off with warm water after 15 minutes. Use avocado as the gentlest exfoliator by blending the flesh with a teaspoon of lemon juice and two tablespoons of smooth wheatgerm. Rub onto your face with gentle, circular movements. Rinse off and moisturise. Any one of these avocado recipes will do just as much for your body, but then it becomes an expensive proposition, so dine on the flesh or use it for the face and rub the oily insides of the skin on your limbs and body before a bath or shower.

Other kitchen remedies

Don't forget the kitchen cupboard bathtime beautifiers. A salt and cooking oil rubdown before your bath is the perfect way to smooth and exfoliate your skin. A handful of powdered milk in the water is great for soothing and moisturising. A muslin bag of oatmeal can be used like soap to smooth the skin, and a cup of cider vinegar added to the bath is invaluable for soothing itchy, flaky skin.

EYE BRIGHTENERS

In theory, skins should look their best after we've enjoyed a restful night's sleep. In practice, many of us retain fluid around the eyes overnight and they look baggy rather than bright at the start of a day. Five to ten minutes with one of the following remedies covering them will reduce puffiness:

● Try using the tea bags from your morning 'cuppa' as a compress for tired eyes, but make sure they are well squeezed out, cool or cold and the tea was well-brewed, as under-brewed tea can stain the skin.

● Thin slices of cucumber or cucumber pulp over the eyelids will tone up the area, and cool and soothe tired eyes. Cucumber has a drying, slightly astringent effect, so don't use it if your eye area is dry or mature.

● Other baggy eye reducers are grated raw apple or potato spread on a thin piece of fabric and placed over the eyes, fabric side down.

● For an instant lift, take an ice cube and smooth it over the upper lid and underneath lower lashes, taking it upwards at the outer corners to the temples. You can use this method about two or three times a week. If your eye area is dry or mature, stick to the gentler tea bag remedy.

● If you are feeling the strain after hours of close encounter with a book, typewriter or VDU screen, take your pick from one of the above remedies and try this relaxer afterwards (or you can use it on its own):
Sit back in your chair and try to quieten your mind for a minute or two. Then, rub the palms of your hands together very quickly about thirty times so that they get quite warm. Take in a deep breath, and cover each eye with a warm palm while you hold your breath for as long as comfortably possible. Slowly release your breath and remove your hands. The combination of heat and total darkness is very relaxing. Repeat two or three times if possible.

PROFESSIONAL TREATMENTS FOR THE SKIN

There still seems to be some strong streak of puritanism in Great Britain about having salon treatments, and many people still believe that it's an area largely for the rich, leisured and self-indulgent. Maybe there should be a change of job title with the word 'beauty' giving way to skin care and health, as so much of the work of therapists is geared towards this area.

Professional treatments for the skin can be divided into two sections: *corrective treatments* (increasingly being recommended by dermatologists) where, a good therapist for instance can help to keep the skin clean, control oil, remove blackheads and whiteheads and help to prevent major eruptions and possible scarring, and *maintenance treatments*, which are designed to cleanse, tone, and firm and bring health and vitality to the skin, relax your body and make you feel better about yourself.

It's not vain to want to look and feel your best and if you have a limited amount of money to spend, it's often wise to choose an appropriate skin or body treatment (plus a good haircut) over a new outfit. Looking and feeling good about yourself gives you that lively, positive look that can help you carry ageing, chain store clothes into loftier realms.

Men should not think that they are excluded from the professional treatments. Increasingly therapists and salons are taking on male clients, and there's certainly a lot they can do for male health and looks, too.

So, if you're new to the beauty treatment business, here are some introductions to professional skin and body improvers.

FACIALS

Facials are one of the most rewarding forms of beauty treatment – partly because your face is so much on show and partly because facials are enjoyable and relaxing. Massage and treatment includes the neck and chest, usually the shoulders, sometimes the back and even the scalp.

Facials generally cleanse, tone, stimulate local circulation and improve skin texture. Depending on your needs, the products and techniques used, they can help control excess oil, remove blackheads, open up and remove whiteheads and improve blemished skin, get reasonable skin working at optimum level and help dried out, mature skin to function more efficiently, and add to its hydration levels. While facials don't remove wrinkles, they do help to make dried-out, tense or mature skins look younger and livelier by easing tension or fine, dry lines.

As there are so many different facials, some devised and given a trade name by the firms involved, it would be difficult and repetitive to mention them individually. Your therapist will tell you about the type(s) she and her salon offer that will be most suitable and rewarding for your skin. There will be minor variations in massage techniques and products applied, and whether the treatment is entirely manual or includes machines, but you are likely to experience the following:

- Your face is carefully examined to discover skin type and possible problems, then cleansed and toned so that work can start on an oil-free skin.

- The face may be steamed to encourage elimination of toxins, dilate pores, and encourage impurities to come to the surface, and aid the application of products. (Incidentally this is a great help if you have a touch of sinus or are suffering from the tail end of a head cold.)

- Most full facials will include exfoliation with a product that will remove any trace of leftover debris and hasten the fall of dead surface cells so that the skin is smooth and fresh.

- If the skin is blemished, manual extraction will be done to remove blackheads and open blocked surfaces of whiteheads.

- After the total cleansing session, the skin will be massaged with anti-bacterial agents, creams, oils or serums according to skin type or the particular facial. This might be done with machines using high frequency or galvanic current to further cleanse the skin, or alternatively, vacuum suction with tiny plastic cups is used in some facials to alleviate puffiness and reduce water retention. Manual massage includes a variety of methods and moves such as stroking, gentle pressure and tapping with fingers. Some massage works on acupressure points, others towards the lymph glands. Whatever the techniques involved, this is the deeply relaxing part of a facial and is followed by a mask which is left on for some minutes while you dream away with your eyes lightly covered to make it even more relaxing.

- The final step is usually the application of some form of firming or moisturising gel, serum or cream.

- While a facial will certainly improve your skin, it may not do so immediately. Short-term blemishes may appear as the skin continues to clear its impurities, so it's wise to have a facial several days before any special occasion, not just the day before.

- Some salons do mini facials which consist of deep cleansing, toning, exfoliation and moisturising. The results are very good, but these take about half as long as a full facial and the session is, naturally, not quite so relaxing.

MAKE-UP LESSONS

Make-up lessons must come into the category of skin enhancers and are certainly rewarding and often money-saving. They can stop you making expensive mistakes with wrong cosmetic buys and are good for someone just starting to wear make-up, who is unsure about colours or techniques of application that suit.

Make-up lessons are also invaluable if you've been wearing the same look for years and it's desperately in need of updating. Or if you want some advice about make-up for a special occasion, such as a wedding. Apart from being shown how to apply foundation, powder, blusher, eye make-up and lipstick and how to choose the best colours to suit you, you will be shown the professional methods of cleansing and moisturising.

Some specialised 'face places' stock many ranges of skin care products and cosmetics and will help you choose and use a range and colours that suit your skin and looks *and* the amount of money you can afford to spend on cosmetics. Some therapists or make-up artists will make you up fully with your new look, whilst others will apply a little of each product and supervise you finishing off each step of the make-up. Others may make up half your face and assist while you make up the other half. Many will give you details of the techniques, products and colours used, but do take notes yourself, and ask questions if you're not sure of anything. Certainly speak up if there's anything you're not too keen on. A cleansing and make-up lesson will take about an hour.

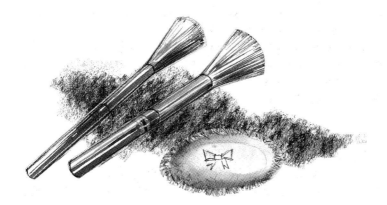

HEAT TREATMENTS

Many forms of heat treatment are used to deep cleanse the skin and stimulate circulation, and are generally very relaxing.

Steam cabinets

These are upright cabinets that you sit in while moist heat circulates around your body. It's like having your own individual Turkish bath with the advantage that your head is outside the steam and this may make you feel less hot and less claustrophobic. Generally the time in the cabinet is 15 minutes, followed by body treatments or a cool shower.

Saunas

Saunas found in swimming baths and gyms are frequently mis-used. Do read and follow the instructions if you're not being supervised. The modern version is usually a specially built wooden room with slatted benches which you sit or lie upon while electric 'coals' give off intense dry heat. Sessions in the heat are usually alternated with cool or cold showers. The Scandinavians have used 'hot sheds' alternated with plunging in the snow as an age-old cure for many ailments and for toning up the body. Cold water stimulates the circulation and energy levels and you'll feel tingling and warm afterwards.

Infra red lamps

These lamps warm and relax the body (as well as relieving painful muscles and joints) and may be used to prepare the body for further treatments or to encourage the penetration of oils.

Heat wrapping

Heat wrapping may be used to cleanse the skin, stimulate circulation, and aid in the removal of waste products. You may lose a little weight during a session, but this is usually replaced as soon as you drink some liquids, so these cannot be considered long-term slimming treatments. There are several forms of treatment where mud, gels, creams, or essential oils are applied and often covered with a body wrapping, a blanket or insulated, waterproof covering while you 'sweat it out'.

Paraffin wax

This cleanses, softens and oils the skin and is a form of heat wrapping where the skin is coated with warm, melted wax and wrapped in foil or blankets for fifteen to thirty minutes. After treatment, the cooled, set wax is peeled off. This treatment can also be used on the hands as part of a manicure or on the face as part of a skin conditioning treatment.

BODY MASSAGE

Body massage stimulates circulation and relaxes tense muscles. It may be used in conjunction with dieting and exercise in a body toning programme. It certainly softens and smooths your skin and helps your body and mind to unwind or re-energise depending upon the type of massage given. It may be done on the entire body, or on parts which often hold tension such as the back and shoulders.

Electrically operated massage machines

Massage machines such as a 'G5' which has different gyratory attachments ranging from hard and knobbly to soft and spongy, may be used on different parts of the body. Machine massage is faster and possibly deeper than hand massage, but more impersonal and less relaxing.

Hand massage

This can be done with specially blended massage oils (which should have a vegetable base) which will allow the therapist's hands to slide and glide more easily, or essential oils which will give extra benefit to the skin and body. You can have a dozen different massages done by a dozen different and first class masseurs or masseuses and all will have developed their own special moves and amount of pressure (although they will usually check on whether you prefer deep or light massage and if you are comfortable and happy at various times during the massage). Any massage is likely to include some or all of the following moves: **effleurage** – calming, warming, stroking movements which stimulate circulation and relax muscles and will probably start and finish the massage, **petrissage** – a deeper, kneading movement for tense muscles, **tapotement** which may be either cupping – where cupped hands move alternately and swiftly over an area or hacking – using the sides of the fingers to stimulate and invigorate the body. In addition, there may be various pressure movements made with the thumb or finger pads on certain points or muscles to work on tense areas or to stimulate circulation. A full body massage will take an hour or so; a back and shoulder massage half an hour.

AROMATHERAPY

True aromatherapy is a total treatment of the face and body via the skin. It alleviates many health troubles such as insomnia, toxic retention, tension, menstrual and menopausal problems and helps your body to achieve a healthy, natural balance. It can certainly improve all skin problems from young and blemished to dry and atrophied. Along the way it makes you feel relaxed, or stimulated depending upon your needs and the oils used. It is certainly a very luxurious and deeply satisfying therapy.

Essential oils

The essential oils used in aromatherapy are a vital part of the treatment. They are obtained, often in minute quantities, from flowers, leaves, roots, berries, seeds, bark and resin and all have some degree of antibiotic, anti-septic and anti-inflammatory properties as well as their specifically stated ones. It is possible to use these oils on yourself, but they are powerful products and this should be done only with advice from your therapist.

While your aromatherapist may have her own blends of essential oils to relax, stimulate or de-toxify according to your needs, here is a resumé of some that are particularly good for a variety of skin conditions:

Benzoin   Benzoin is calming, and sedative. It is used for certain skin irritations and pigmentation problems and also for arthritis and respiratory disorders.

Bergamot   Bergamot is often used where there is acne. It is also good for feverish infections and depression. (Avoid strong UV rays for 48 hours after using or you'll risk pigmentation problems.)

Camomile   Camomile is soothing. Helps with inflammation in eczema, sunburn, allergies, acne, and aids skin healing. It also encourages sound sleep.

Cedarwood   Cedarwood can help with a variety of skin problems and ailments and is also good for the respiratory system.

Cypress   Cypress is good for acne and associated problems, dehydrated skins and broken veins.

Eucalyptus   Eucalyptus is well-known as an aid to respiratory problems and it also helps skin heal.

Geranium   Geranium aids circulation and healing, and is good for sensitive skins.

Juniper   Juniper is used to cleanse and detoxify, and is good for acne. It also helps reduce tension.

Lavender   Lavender is one of the most used oils and is excellent for most skin conditions.

Lemongrass   Lemongrass is great for oily, disturbed skin.

Myrrh   Myrrh is used for blemished, inflamed skin.

Neroli   Neroli is anti-bacterial, mildly hypnotic. It is much used for skin care and sleeping problems.

Patchouli   Patchouli is very soothing and much used in skin care.

Peppermint   Peppermint is also very soothing, used for skin irritations, bruising, and sprains.

Rose   Rose is excellent for most skin types, particularly dry mature and sensitive ones.

Rosemary   Rosemary is used in skin care, particularly when there is fluid retention.

Sage   Sage is a good balancer for oily or devitalised skin.

Sandalwood   Sandalwood revitalises dry and dehydrated skins.

Ylang-ylang   Ylang-ylang is great for general care of the skin and it's also said to be an aphrodisiac.

Aromatherapy massage

Aromatherapy massage is based on ancient Chinese massage of the connective tissue and lymph drainage. It is quite unlike Swedish massage taught during basic training, although, an aromatherapist will have been trained in beauty therapy or may have been a nurse, and will display a certificate showing she has been further trained in aromatherapy. Massage will be gentle and soothing and follow these general moves:

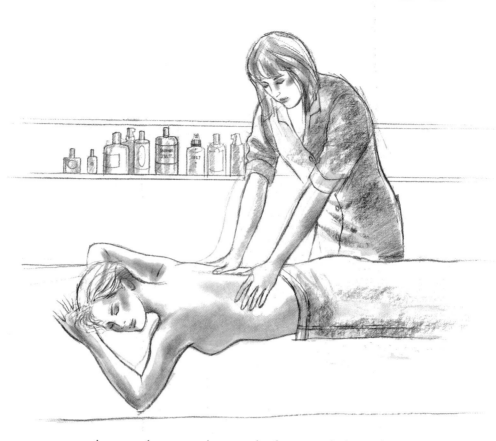

An aromatherapy session must be the most relaxing and
luxurious treatment you can have.

After questioning you very closely about diet, family background,
medical history and lifestyle (all very relevant) your aromatherapist will
make a close study of your skin (and perhaps your feet) which will indicate
much to her about the state of your health as well as the condition of your
skin.

Massage will start with the backs of the legs and move to the back which
will include 'sounding out' pressure points on either side of the spine. This
indicates the state of health of various organs of your body. There will be
further back massage, including work on the shoulders and neck. The
front of the body, the upper chest and entire abdominal area will be gently
massaged in various ways and at times you may be asked to do breathing
techniques to assist in some of the treatments. Most aromatherapy
treatments include massage of the face (plus a mask) and some the head,
but in all cases massage follows the lymphatic channels and works on
lymph drainage.

Many aromatherapy treatments include reflexology – and a full treatment takes about an hour and a half. It is important that you don't eat for at least 2 hours before the treatment, and that you have light meals for the rest of the day and drink plenty of water (no alcohol or you could develop a splitting headache as treatment detoxifies, and drinking alcohol reintroduces toxins). Don't have any form of heat treatment before the session and keep out of the sun or any form of strong UV rays for 24 hours after treatment.

REFLEXOLOGY

Reflexology is often used at some stage during an aromatherapy treatment. This ancient therapy originated in China thousands of years ago and is based on the belief that there are energy channels or reflexes in the feet corresponding to every part of the body. When a given part of the body is not working perfectly, tiny, crystal-like granules are to be found under the skin of the feet. Moving over the area with thumb or finger pads using strong, but not hard, pressure is painless if the relevant part of the body is in top working order, but can feel like sandpaper if it's less than perfect, and can cause some discomfort if the particular part of the body is not working well. Stroking pressure on any granules relieves the energy channels and the relevant organ or part of the body.

If you've never had this treatment and it all sounds weird and unbelievable, just check, next time you're in a very tense state or have something like 'flu, on just how painful your feet are.

During treatment, it's astounding how a good practitioner will pick up problems you haven't mentioned or, for instance, leap in on your kidney and liver area when you've been wining and dining too well too often or on your adrenal and diaphragm areas on your feet when you're tense and stressed. Despite possible short-term discomfort at times during the session, you will be very relaxed afterwards and should have relief (particularly after a series of treatments) from many conditions that may have caused you a certain amount of suffering.

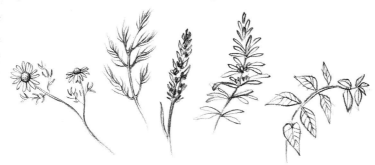

ENJOYING YOUR TREATMENT

Look for the following when you go for treatment:

- The salon and therapist should be clean, neat and organised and the atmosphere friendly, happy and relaxing.

- You should be given a consultation (which is usually free) and explanation of what's involved before having any treatment that's new to you. The therapist will ask you many questions so that she knows a lot about your life, your medical history and your needs. (It's often very relevant to a treatment to find out whether you're stressed, tired, have been unwell recently or are on any sort of medication.)

- The therapist should make and keep a record of you and your treatments and refer to them whenever you visit.

- Find out in advance how much a treatment(s) will cost rather than worry about your possible bill and ruin your relaxation and enjoyment.

- Don't be afraid to ask questions about what's being done, the products used and how you can keep up the good work at home.

- There must be a sympathetic relationship between the two of you for everything to work successfully. Beauty treatments are a very personal experience and a therapist may be first-class and adored by many clients, but if you don't feel completely at ease with her, you won't thoroughly enjoy the treatment.

- On your side of the relationship – be punctual, honest and interested.

- If you've enjoyed your session, feel better and feel you look better, do say so. As with any job, it's good to have a feedback and to know that your work is pleasing.

YOUR GUIDE TO A GOOD THERAPIST

Given a lot of cheek, you or I or any unqualified person could open up a clinic or salon and call ourselves a therapist as at present there is no government supervision of qualifications. You can make sure that your therapist has high qualifications and high standards by making a few checks before making an appointment:

The easiest, quickest and most foolproof method is to look at her qualifying certificates, recognised diplomas in beauty therapy and her insurance. No highly trained therapist will mind you asking, indeed certificates are quite likely to be framed and displayed around the salon.

Training for therapists is intensive and extensive, and is undertaken in technical colleges or private beauty schools where students study every aspect of beauty care from anatomy to practical applications of treatments. Examinations must be passed before they obtain their recognised certificates. The following are the certificates to look for to ensure your face and body are in safe and highly trained hands:

CIBTAC (Confederation of International Beauty Therapy and Cosmetology) – this is the British Association of Beauty Therapy (BABTAC) examination which is held by many private schools and technical colleges.

CIDESCO (Comité International d'Esthetique et de Cosmetologie) – a qualification awarded in private beauty therapy schools and some technical colleges. CIDESCO is an international organisation with schools in many countries.

City and Guilds – a qualification taken mainly by people trained at technical colleges.

ITEC (International Therapy Examination Council) – taken in private schools and technical colleges.

International Health and Beauty Council – This examination is taken in some technical colleges and private beauty schools.

It's an added assurance if your therapist is a member of a professional organisation. This means that her qualifications are recognised, her standards are high and the salon well-maintained and insured against accidents.

BABTAC is the British Association of Beauty Therapy and Cosmetology (which has thousands of members in Britain and will be able to recommend a highly qualified therapist in your area – for their address, see page 171).

The Society of International Health and Beauty Therapists.

CHAPTER SEVEN

DEALING WITH SKIN PROBLEMS

BEAUTY SPOTS . . . OR MINOR BLEMISHES

Moles may be called beauty spots, and blushing and freckles considered charming. But if they and other small skin problems upset you, they can be made less noticeable with care and cosmetics – and they will often disappear with time or a touch of treatment. Do keep your problems in perspective. Our own faces are magnified by close encounters with a mirror – other people seldom study them as searchingly or caringly as we do.

BLUSHING

Everyone has felt a hot flush of embarrassment coming over them at some time – shy and emotional people suffer this more than most, and fine, pale skins have a greater tendency to show the glow. Given an exciting, nerve-wracking or embarrassing situation, a chain reaction in the body causes dilation of the superficial blood vessels in the dermis and the increased blood flow turns the skin a hot shade of pink. It's a frequent and common occurrence in the young – we've all seen children blush 'to the roots of their hair' when teased. Princess Diana made the process world news when she was younger and newer at her job. Of course, growing older and less vulnerable to public opinion will diminish the blush reaction. You'll really just have to wait for time, age and experience to make its mark if you're a frequent blusher!

BLOTCHING

This arises from a blood flow reaction similar to blushing, but distribution is patchy and often confined to the neck. Again, it's usually a stress response and a degree of emotional control will lower the incidence. If you've not been a flusher and it suddenly comes upon you during the menopause, you can lay the blame on your hormones again. No one quite understands why this happens and you'll be much more aware of it than anyone else. Again, it's a case of waiting for the problem to pass.

CYSTS

Cary Grant had them, de Niro's and Robert Redford's are very obvious, yet they certainly didn't harm their job prospects! There are many types of cyst, and they can contain a fluid or fairly solid substance. They are sometimes reminders of a burnt-out case of acne. If you don't like these small flesh-coloured lumps on your face or body, they can be removed by a dermatologist.

FRECKLES

Freckles are localised melanin deposits. They are usually inherited, and can look very charming. But, freckled skin is delicate, and should be highly protected from UV rays if it's going to look young for as long as possible. Youthful freckled skins look good with just a day covering of tinted moisturiser or you can tone down freckles by using a neutral beige foundation applied with a damp sponge (don't choose a dark shade in an effort to match the freckles – it doesn't work) and translucent powder. Getting rid of freckles is pretty impossible – bleaching creams have little effect and can cause a reaction on delicate skins.

LENTIGINOSES

These are more commonly known as 'liver spots', although they have nothing to do with your liver. These flat, brown, irregular blotches are most often found on hands that have seen forty summers or more and a lot of sun exposure. There's nothing dangerous or even particularly ugly about them, but the age connotation does make them rather unwelcome to some people. They can be frozen or rubbed off by a dermatologist. Use a good sunblock to prevent further arrivals.

MOLES

From Regency fops to present-day film stars – everyone it seems loves the well-placed beauty spot. But if your moles are large, hairy, or madly profuse, they can be an embarrassment. Even if you don't like them, moles are nothing to worry about on health grounds unless they change shape, grow larger, or bleed, in which case you must go for medical advice immediately. (Never poke or pick at a mole yourself.) If necessary, a dermatologist can remove small moles in a matter of minutes under local anaesthetic.

SKIN TAGS

Skin tags are small pieces of excess skin about the size of a grain of rice that usually appear on the neck or under the armpits. They disappear when the blood supply is cut off. A skilled electrolysist can do this job.

OPEN PORES

These are distended hair follicles that have widened to accommodate heavy outpourings of sebum. Scrupulous treatment of an oily skin will minimise their occurrence and an oil-free tinted foundation and matt make-up will make them look less obvious. While it's important to use a toner after cleansing, this will not close or tighten the pores – nothing will.

RED FACE

Redness on the cheeks may be inherited or can belong to a sensitive skin that's been exposed to extremes of weather either hot or cold, without adequate protection. Keep the colour under control by avoiding very hot drinks, alcohol, hot and spicy foods, and protect your skin from strong winds, hot sun and icy weather. Women can tone down the high colour with a neutral shade of foundation.

SALLOW SKIN

This skin type usually belongs to people with Mediterranean looks – dark hair, dark eyes and olive skin – after they've faced a long British winter. Exercise and fresh air at all times of the year will give this skin a healthier look and will improve circulation. Use a complexion brush when you wash your face, and massage movements when you use a cleansing lotion. Don't try to warm your looks with a pinky shade of foundation. A neutral beige is

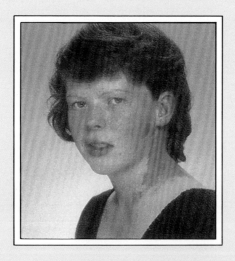

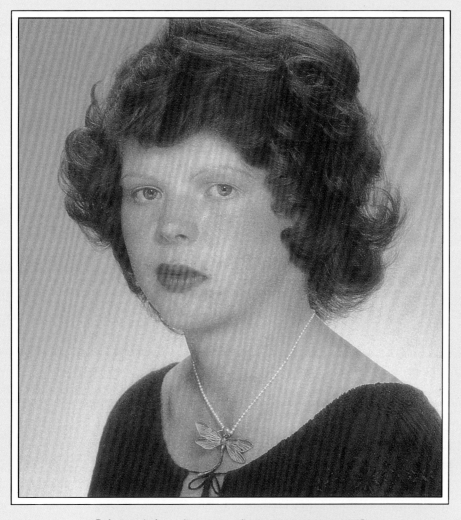

Before and after using a camouflage cream (see page 145).

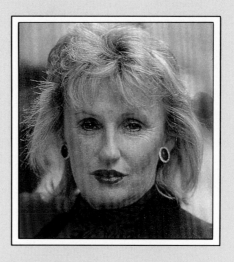

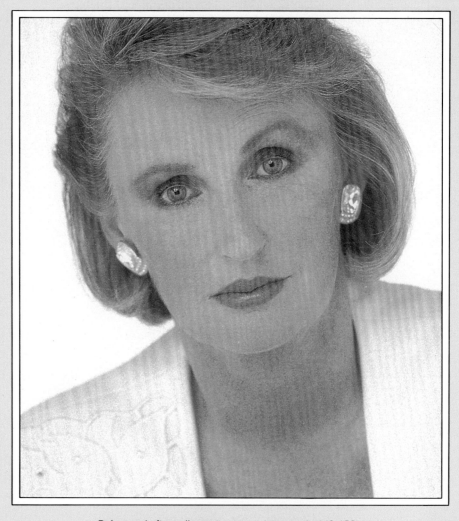

Before and after collagen treatment (see pages 149-150).

best, topped with translucent powder and blusher on cheeks. Finish with the lightest flick of the blusher brush over forehead, nose and jawline.

THREAD VEINS

Thread veins, red veins, broken veins, call them what you like (the medical term is *Telangiectases*), but those tiny red veins often found on the cheeks are caused by dilation of the capillaries in the dermis. They can be an inherited condition, and tend to appear on fine, sensitive skin. It's wise to treat them gently, and avoid extremes of heat and cold in food, drink, weather and facial treatments. Thread veins are often treated very successfully with diathermy to cauterise the capillaries. Done by a skilled electrolysist, who is qualified to work on these veins, this is a relatively minor treatment and any discoloration disappears in a matter of days.

MORE SERIOUS SKIN PROBLEMS

While skin takes a miraculous amount of punishment and usually springs back into form, there are common problems that need varying degrees of help according to their severity. While it would take a medical encyclopaedia to cover all skin ailments, here are some common ones.

ACNE

Acne is certainly not only a teenage trouble, but because spots, eruptions and acne are a plague at puberty, it's dealt with in detail in chapter 3.

ALLERGIES

When your body disapproves of or disagrees with a substance that's put on or inside it, it releases a chemical called *histamine* (which is why some allergies are sometimes treated with substances termed *anti-histamines*) and this leads to the symptoms we recognise as an allergy. These can include rashes, blotches, swelling on the skin, nausea, and many more distressing symptoms depending upon the strength of reaction.

Perfumes, toiletries, hair dyes and cosmetics are a possible source of allergens, and so are preservatives and dyes in foods, household cleansers, detergents, garden products, animal hair and household dust. There is no end to the possible culprits. Reaction is always more likely or more violent when you are under stress, and make-up and perfumes you normally wear with joy can, when they're worn in the sun, induce phototoxic or photoallergenic reactions. Of course, it's easier to identify the allergen if reaction is around the contact area – for instance on your hands when you've recently dipped them in a new brand of detergent – but it can take time for the symptoms to appear, and they don't always crop up where contact is obvious. Some time ago, a spate of problems around the eye area was traced to an ingredient in nail polish. Just think how often you touch your eyes with your hands. If you're inclined to allergies, opt for hypoallergenic cosmetics which are screened to be free from all known irritants.

If you can identify the substance your body doesn't like, avoid it. If you have suspicions, do your own patch test by putting a little of the product on the soft skin inside your elbow, covering it with a plaster, and leaving it for twenty-four hours. If you're allergic there'll be a red or blotchy mark. When the source is impossible to discover, and reaction is strong, get medical advice.

BIRTHMARKS

Birthmarks are discoloured patches of skin caused by flaws in the development of blood vessels or pigment distribution before birth. The raised *strawberry birthmark* usually fades or disappears before puberty. *Port wine stains*, which look as though ruby-red port has been spilt on the skin, don't. Your doctor will advise you whether a birthmark is likely to fade, and will suggest treatment for more extensive and obvious ones. It is sometimes possible to have them removed with dermabrasion, laser treatment or a skin graft. Birthmarks can be covered very successfully with camouflage treatment.

BITES AND STINGS

The odd mosquito, wasp or bee sting can be uncomfortable or painful, but treatment with a piece of ice, a sting-calming product or calamine lotion will alleviate discomfort and they should be no problem unless they become infected through scratching or you have an allergy to the sting. A host of them can cause real trouble – even one wasp landing on a lolly as it reaches your child's mouth can be tricky. If you're worried or if there's a nasty reaction, get your doctor's advice. Dog, cat and snake bites and a severe clash with several jellyfish when you're swimming will require medical attention.

BLISTERS

Pressure, rubbing and suction cause a build-up of fluid or blood under the skin (a love bite is in fact a blood blister). Remove the source of irritation (or the passionate partner), and leave the blister alone, or cover it to prevent further pressure, and it will go away.

BOILS

Boils are major-league infected spots that are often yet another skin problem at puberty. Keep them scrupulously clean, and treat them with warm compresses – made from clean cotton wool wrung out in hot water. If they don't burst within a matter of days, and you have a spate of them or one in an awkward place such as on your buttocks, see a doctor. Antibiotics may be prescribed.

BRUISES

These are caused by a collection of blood under the skin where a knock or blow has fractured blood vessels. The blood pigment is gradually absorbed by the body with the surface of the affected skin turning to rainbow hues before returning to normal. If you're inclined to rush around bashing your body in the process or play body contact games or bruise very easily, make sure your diet is rich in vitamin C which helps maintain healthy blood vessels. Eat plenty of fresh (preferably uncooked) green vegetables and salads, potatoes, citrus fruits, tomatoes, apricots, cherries, grapes and strawberries. If you're not sure of the freshness of your fruit and vegetables, take a vitamin C supplement daily.

BURNS

Burns can be caused by fire, certain chemicals, hot liquids and fats. Painful, red skin from sunburn (or any other source) constitutes *first degree* burns; *second degree* burns bring pain, redness and blistering; and *third degree* burns affect the full thickness of skin and can leave scars.

In the case of burning, get yourself or the patient immediately away from the source of the burn. Treat the area with cold, running water, but otherwise don't touch it or put anything on it. If the burn is serious, get immediate medical attention.

Superficial burns heal on their own, but deeper ones that have caused scarring can be treated with skin grafts. (Falklands hero Simon Weston is an example of incredible skin reconstruction and plastic surgery.)

CANCER OF THE SKIN

Skin cancer is common in parts of the world where there's a lot of hot sunshine. It was once rare in Great Britain, but is increasing rapidly with the trends to greater leisure and holidays in hotter parts of the world.

Any changes in skin texture, moles, scars or the development of rough, raised patches should be examined medically. It's likely to be a false alarm, but it's always better to be safe than sick. There are many types of skin cancer and with early diagnosis and treatment the chances of a complete cure are high.

CHLOASMA

Chloasma is a pigmentation problem causing patches of darker colour on the skin. It's often associated with pregnancy and the contraceptive pill, and usually fades within a matter of months of having the baby or coming off the Pill. In the meantime, cover up under the sun, wear a sunblock, and a hat – the sun makes the darker patches an even stronger shade.

COLD SORES

Cold sores are caused by a virus and tend to appear when the skin is sensitised by a body infection, stress or sunshine. Prickling blisters appear, often around the mouth and nostrils and develop into nasty, watery sores. They are infectious and can be passed on via towels, crockery and kissing. Surgical spirit or cologne helps dry the blisters out, and you can buy specific products for this problem at chemists and health shops. I swear by the following tip which was given to me by a make-up artist – apply damp, used coffee grounds, or instant coffee dampened with a drop of water, on the cold sore and leave it for ten minutes before rinsing off with warm water. This takes away the discomfort and swelling and speeds the healing process.

DERMATITIS

Dermatitis means inflammation of the skin and the term is almost interchangeable with Eczema (see below).

ECZEMA

Eczema is a non-contagious skin condition typified by dry, scaly, itchy, inflamed and often sore, blistered, weeping and bloody skin which can cause physical and mental distress to the sufferer, and to whole families, particularly where a baby or small child is concerned. There are many types of eczema, but the upsetting and often desperately uncomfortable symptoms may be similar and it is important to consult a GP or specialist for precise diagnosis and help. It is estimated that one in ten people suffer from some form of eczema during their lives.

Contact dermatitis or eczema
This problem is caused by direct irritants (when the site of the rash and the speed of reaction is likely to indicate the cause) such as soaps, washing powders and solvents. *Allergic contact dermatitis* occurs when a body develops a sudden allergy to substances it has previously been harmlessly in contact with, perhaps for years – anything from metals and jewellery to certain toiletries, cosmetics or materials handled at work.

Atopic eczema
This is the most common form of eczema and can be connected with contact, eating or inhaling a wide range of substances to which the particular body is allergic. While cause and cure are still subject to conjecture, it is believed to be the result of an imbalance in the immune system which is over-zealous and reacts too strongly to a wide range of stimuli. There is a hereditary predisposition to atopic eczema and in many cases there may be a family history of hay fever or asthma. It is largely a disease of babies, children and young people, but it can continue into adult life.

Seborrhoeic eczema
This form of eczema can be confused with atopic eczema, but it usually only affects babies and adults (particularly men) from their twenties to forties and is usually worse on the scalp, but can spread to the face and body, especially the groin and armpits.

Discoid eczema
Discoid eczema takes the form of scaly, itchy, round-shaped patches found on the limbs.

Varicose eczema
Varicose eczema is common in the elderly, when skin becomes drier, and in people suffering from varicose veins. Other types of eczema can affect older people, and it is thought they are the result of a constitutional dispo-

sition to develop the condition which is then triggered by the fact that the workings of the body are less efficient with age.

It is clear that eczema can strike at any time in life. Stress usually increases the problem, and so does overheating (caused by central heating, very hot weather or excessive clothing). Humidity, hard water, cigarette smoke and other irritants such as certain fabrics, household dust and washing powders can add to the problem. The list of possible triggers is endless. Of course, the extreme irritation, the unbearable itching and consequent scratching can lead to infection.

While there is as yet no cure, medication and practical steps can be taken to help keep eczema under control and make life more bearable. Diet can help in some cases, and emollients and the sparing use of steroid ointments may be prescribed to combat the skin condition. Antihistamines may be prescribed to act as a sedative and help with sleep. Oil of Evening Primrose is being used with success by some patients; others have found help through alternative therapies, and doctors and dermatologists are now beginning to work with alternative therapists including a current study on the benefits of Chinese herbal medicine.

The National Eczema Society provides back-up help for members and non-members with an information service, leaflets (including in six Asian languages) and information packs containing dos and don'ts of skin care and how to cope with all aspects of eczema. There are different packs relating to babies and children, teenagers and adults. The Society helps to fund research into finding causes, cures and better methods of management for people living with this problem.

IMPETIGO

Impetigo is caused by an infection, and manifests as watery blisters that develop into scabby, weeping sores. It spreads quickly and is contagious. The condition responds to antibiotics and treatment should be started as soon as possible.

PLANTAR WARTS

Plantar warts are also known as verrucae. They are foot warts which are easily contracted in sports changing rooms and swimming baths. Walking on them can be painful. Your pharmacist or doctor will suggest treatment although they sometimes disappear of their own accord (like any wart).

Never cut or dig at them yourself. Cover them with plasters (or rubber shoes when you're swimming) to avoid passing them on to others.

PSORIASIS

Psoriasis is a non-contagious skin disorder typified by raised red patches covered with silvery scales. The turnover of epidermal cells goes haywire, and instead of taking the normal three to four weeks to shed the top layer of skin, psoriasis sufferers can take three to four days, so both live and dead cells can accumulate on the surface in a visible, chaotic layer. Well over a million people in the UK and something like 80 million throughout the world suffer from it – from relatively mild, contained patches that come and go (but can still be a source of embarrassment and discomfort at times) to thankfully rare, devastating cases where the whole body is affected (like the hero in Dennis Potter's TV serial, *The Singing Detective*). Psoriasis may first appear at any age, but the most frequent starting point is some time between puberty and middle age. It does run in families, but it seems that a genetic tendency can be triggered by physical and emotional stress, skin injury, throat infections and certain drugs. At least one third of psoriatics lose the condition naturally for long periods of time or even for good. Certainly happy, fresh-air holidays and relaxation help improve the obvious condition in most cases (this is one of the reasons why hypnosis, self-hypnosis and any relaxing techniques can be a good idea).

The exact causes of and permanent cure for this condition are not yet known, but many cases are controlled or improved by a variety of treatments including taking brewer's yeast, fish oils or Oil of Evening Primrose. Medically controlled doses of UVA and UVB rays are used with some success and surface treatments include coal tars, dithranol and Dovonex – a derivative of vitamin D. Research is being carried out into the genetic aspects of psoriasis and skin biopsies of HIV patients are being used to attempt to find out more about psoriasis in HIV and non-HIV patients.

The Psoriasis Association provides a point of social contact for sufferers, advances education for people with psoriasis and the general public (to increase understanding and acceptance) and collects funds for research projects.

SCARS

When severely cut or damaged, skin rarely heals invisibly. Collagen/elastin bundles become denser, blood vessels, hair follicles, sweat glands may be destroyed, the surrounding skin becomes taut and the surface of the scar tissue become red or white from loss of melanin. Afro-Caribbeans and Orientals (and Caucasians with vigorously healing skin) are prone to keloids – thickened scar tissue – and darker or lighter pigmentation at the scar site. Keeping the skin moisturised will help the appearance of taut skin around a scar. Cosmetic camouflage can help with looks as can various treatments by a plastic surgeon if the scar is obvious and causing distress.

STRETCH MARKS

These are the result of scar tissue just beneath the skin's surface, caused by stretch and strain over a period of time. They are associated with hormone changes in the body. Initially red or purple, the colour fades and they become white or silvery. They can occur at puberty, but are commonly associated with pregnancy or when someone has been very overweight. Most common sites are the pelvic area and breasts. They're a permanent fixture once they happen. Prevent them as much as possible by not becoming overweight or putting on more weight than your doctor or clinic advise when you're pregnant. While it will not necessarily prevent stretch marks oiling the skin to keep it as supple as possible is a good idea. As long as your body's in good shape, wear your bikini and be damned.

TATTOOS

Tattoos are a self-chosen skin affliction that these days must fall into the category of plain madness. Pigment is introduced into the skin by needles – with the consequent risk of infection and the spreading of blood related diseases. Tattoos are there for life, barring some radical treatment such as removal by laser or surgery.

VAGINAL THRUSH

Vaginal thrush is a fungus infection of the mucous membranes caused by a slight breakdown in the body's natural defence organisms. Happening in this area, the irritation it can cause is distressing and embarrassing, and the condition can be passed on through close sexual encounters. Thrush thrives in warm, moist conditions and tights, nylon pants, and body-hugging trousers help it to flourish. Other possible culprits are menstruation, the contraceptive pill, pregnancy, menopause, antibiotics, bath additives, and being tired and stressed. Keep the area as cool as possible, and wear baggy pants, and cotton underclothes. You should also drink plenty of water, eat live yoghurt, add half a cupful of cider vinegar to your bath water and apply live yoghurt to the area to help restore healthy vaginal flora. Put some yoghurt on a tampon for internal treatment. Seek medical advice if it doesn't clear up quickly.

VITILIGO

Vitiligo is loss of pigment in sharply defined areas giving a piebald effect which is particularly obvious on dark-skinned people and is emphasised by a suntan. Do get medical advice, although the cause and cure for vitiligo are unknown at the moment. In visible areas, the contrast between dark and light patches can be diminished with camouflage make-up. Use high SPF products to protect areas lacking pigment.

WARTS

Warts are caused by a virus. They are an overgrowth of skin cells and can be transmitted to other parts of your body or to other people by contact. They may disappear on their own accord and can be removed by chemicals (ask your pharmacist) or mechanical means (by a dermatologist).

DEALING WITH SUPERFLUOUS HAIR

A man can be hairy as a bear and love it – and be loved. For a woman, hair where she doesn't want it can spoil her lifestyle, and her life, even if the problem is more obvious to her eyes than to other people's. If you're a fairly hairy female and you don't care, that's fine. But, if you dread the summer strip off, and hesitate to drop into a dress shop on the spur of the moment or are currently mumbling behind your hand as you cover your moustache, do something about it. You can! Words like 'down' and 'defuzzing' don't seem to apply, do they? So I promise I'll call hair by its real name – hair!

If you clam up about the subject, and refuse to discuss it, even with a great friend or the man you've lived with and loved for years, the problem can loom large and depressingly in your life. Talking takes the taboo out of it – it may help you to find a good beauty therapist or electrolysist someone has been to with great success. But if you're just starting to tackle the problem, here's help on how to do it properly, plus warnings about the methods you should avoid.

BLEACHING

This treatment is great if the hair is fine. Gentle bleaching creams that can be bought from most chemists do a good job. But, a heavy-ish, dark growth can show up more when it's turned to a shade of orange by bleaching with peroxide. Keep bleaching to facial hair if it's not too coarse or dark and arms which are very much in view when they're bare. Removal of hair from these areas by any method other than electrolysis is not a good idea. Bleaching can affect darkly pigmented skins.

SHAVING

Shaving is fast, cheap, convenient and okay for some areas. But, regrowth is immediate and cut ends are blunt instead of tapered, so hair will appear to be thicker (it isn't), feel bristly and, as it hasn't had any bleaching from sun exposure, is likely to be darker. Take your time, and use an electric razor or shaving cream and a safety razor or you could end up with some nasty nicks. You can shave areas like underarms, legs from the knee down, and the bikini line as long as overspill doesn't extend down the thighs.

ABRASIVE PADS

Abrasive mitts or pads gently rub away the hair. They're safe, easy to use, and more aesthetically pleasing than shaving, which smacks of the male morning chore. Although the results are as short term as razor work, they do seem to get closer to the skin and leave it feeling softer for a very short time. Use them only on legs from the knee down.

DEPILATORY CREAMS

Depilatories dissolve the hair by chemical reaction. The very short term results are again better than shaving, but the hair grows back immediately. These products can upset some skins, so do a patch test first. Use on underarms, lower legs and bikini line. Don't use them on the arms or face unless you're desperate and can't afford electrolysis. Again, this can affect darkly pigmented skins.

TWEEZING AND CUTTING

Cut mole hairs and the more obvious ones that pop up between electrolysis sessions but leave the rest well alone. Tweezing is for your eyebrows only.

Plucking hair distorts the follicle, and can make subsequent electrolysis and waxing more tricky.

PLUCKING MACHINES

Electrically operated 'plucking machines' that look something like a razor, but pull out complete hairs have come on to the market in recent years. They are not quite as efficient as a good wax job, but they will soon pay their way if they take the place of salon waxing. Some people can't stand the discomfort, but this is minimised as you get used to the sensation and relax, so you're not working on a tense body. They're not bulky, so can be taken and used in most parts of the world when you're travelling. They're good for legs from the knee down and backs of thighs and results last as long as waxing.

WAXING

Waxing rips out the complete hair – and is basically a form of mass plucking. The treated area stays smooth for around three weeks and regrowth is usually progressively weaker. It can be a little painful, particularly if you're feeling tense. Other drawbacks are that the hair has to be long enough – and therefore visible – to be caught up in the wax and regrowth doesn't always come smoothly through the follicles, so there can be a few bumps as hairs try to break through the skin.

There are several methods of waxing including kits for home use, but DIY wax work can be messy, nerve wracking, and painful if you're a novice. It's more luxurious and usually better done by a good beauty therapist. Waxing is first class for legs, underarms and peripheral pubic hair. It can be used for the face and arms, but it's an 'everything goes' method that takes off fine hairs as well as coarse. And regrowth has to be a certain length (and showing) before wax will take up hairs and remove them. Don't go in the sun for a couple of days after waxing, as it can lead to pigmentation problems.

ORGANIC WAX

This product looks and spreads like honey and works in the same way as wax by lifting out the whole hair including that from below the surface, so re-growth takes weeks to appear. The difference is in the composition of the stripper which is made from 'natural' ingredients – fructose, saccharose, citric acid and water – which may be better for some skins, and spills or patches left on the skin are easily washed away with warm water.

THREADING

Threading is an ancient and highly specialised Oriental method of removing hair using a piece of cotton thread twisted around a finger, so it picks up the hairs that are showing and pulls out the entire hair including what's growing below the surface. Re-growth doesn't appear for some weeks and eventually becomes weaker. The advantages over wax are: very small strips are worked on at a time and hairs are always removed whole with no breaking off at the surface, no products are applied to the skin (to which it could be allergic) and the skin is not stretched in the process, so it is suitable for delicate areas such as the face. It also avoids the risk of pigmentation patches, so is very suitable for darker skins. Best for facial hair and fine hair on arms.

ELECTROLYSIS

The good news is that electrolysis can permanently remove superfluous hair. But don't expect an instant miracle. It takes time and money – just how much of both depends on many factors, including how extensive and heavy the growth and whether previous plucking or waxing have distorted the hair follicle. The entire situation will be discussed on your first visit, but don't expect any electrolysist to be able to tell you exactly just how many visits you'll need straight away.

Hairs are removed one at a time, so it's quite a slow process. Time, expense and cosmetic factors mean electrolysis is most often used for the face, but a good electrolysist can and probably has worked practically everywhere on the face and body. Never be shy of discussing your particular problem with her and finding out if she can resolve it.

For years, the most widely used method of permanent hair removal in Great Britain has been Short Wave or RF diathermy. This is a *radio wave* electric current of *minute proportion* which is introduced into the hair follicle for a second via a very fine needle. The precise current coagulates the papilla (the hair's source of nourishment) which is at the base of the follicle and the hair is loosened and lifted out with tweezers. Treated hairs may grow again if the generative tissue is not completely destroyed, but the structure is weakened with each treatment and eventually disappears for good.

The popularity of the RF method is due to its relatively quick application compared to the galvanic treatment (which uses a chemical reaction – hence the naming of the original method electrolysis). If both currents are very precisely *blended* together the treatment is potentially far more effective – utilising the best effects of each method. But, introduction of this method in the UK is recent and reflects current technology advances.

Pioneering electrolysist Rita Roberts has practised for over thirty years, working with all these methods before developing the latest technology – the *Digital Blend System*. This offers highly efficient treatment for areas of hair growth which are normally considered 'difficult' – for example the neck, underarms, bikini line – where follicles are often curved and hair type is resistant. The precise and programmed *blending* of the Digital Blend currents is assisted by a follicle moisture reading of each hair which helps determine the most appropriate treatment selection.

Many experienced operators now work with both RF and the Blend method to offer their clients greater treatment choice.

The sensation of electrolysis is best described as a tingling feeling – although some areas and skin are extra sensitive and everyone can find a little discomfort where there are more nerve endings – the centre of the upper lip, near the pubic region and stomach area. Skin reaction on all but the sensitive is rarely more than a slight redness and some operators may choose to use an insulated needle for RF treatment to minimise reddening. An initial patch test will help assess individual reaction to treatment.

If you are worried about the possibility of transmittable diseases from treatment, be assured. All electrolysis needles are pre-sterilized and disposable. All premises in which electrolysis is given must register with the local authority whose health inspectors enforce rigid standards of hygiene and sterility.

It is vital that your electrolysist is properly trained and asking to see proof of qualifications (if not displayed) is your prerogative. There are two organisations which represent the specialist electrolysist: The British Association of Electrolysists and The Institute of Electrolysists. Both of these professional bodies demand rigorous training standards and practical salon experience before operators can register as full members. The letters MBAE or FBAE acknowledge British Association membership, the letters DRE (Diploma in Remedial Electrolysis) full membership of the Institute. Both organisations provide an address list of their membership.

While a poorly trained operator can lead clients to disillusionment at best and scarring at worst, just imagine what you could do to yourself. Do *not* buy or use DIY electrolysis kits. Even an expert with a professional machine would hesitate to work on herself – an amateur can cause real and distressing problems.

Electrolygist, electrolysist, electro-therapist all describe the same skill and professional who operates the electrolysis machine.

Superfluous hair facts

- A fine growth of downy (vellus) hair is perfectly normal, and should be left where it grows. This is not superfluous hair. But some people have coarser and/or darker hair than others – it's all in those genes.

- Fine hairs can sometimes coarsen as a result of hormone upheavals, for example during puberty, pregnancy, or the menopause, or after a hysterectomy.

- Women in high pressure jobs have been found to have increased facial hair. It's not a question of a woman being more like a man in every way, but rather that stress can serve to stimulate the hormones.

- Sunshine is taking a real battering. Electrolysists find that female sun worshippers sometimes develop coarser hairs on their face and body.

- Some medically prescribed drugs for very serious illnesses can encourage coarser hair growth (your doctor will worn you of the possibility) and so can certain glandular-affecting illnesses like anorexia.

- Electrolysis treatment is provided through the dermatology department of some NHS hospitals, so GPs are able to refer their patients for this form of treatment. But the GP's decision to refer a patient, and the decision to do electrolysis or not, depends on many clinical factors. It is not simply a matter of the severity of the condition.

- Many electrolysists take male clients who want to get rid of *their* superfluous hair, particularly on cheeks, nose and between the eyebrows.

COSMETIC COVER-UPS

THE BARBARA DALY DISGUISE

It's one of life's beauty ironies that your skin can be perfect when nothing interesting is happening in your life, and look dreadful when something important is in the offing. Excitement, tension and a little jiggling of the hormones don't help. When you want to look good, and your skin doesn't, who better to come to the rescue than Barbara Daly, top make-up artist and creator of Colourings at the Body Shop? Here's her advice:

'Nobody's face is flawless, and concealer is a magical piece of make-up. Choose a shade which will blend in with your skin tone, and use a lip or eyeshadow brush loaded up from the stick just as you would if you were going to put on lipstick.

'Put the concealer on the back of your hand and work from there. The warmth of your hand helps to soften it, so you don't use too much and you're not dabbing the brush on a spot and back on your concealer stick this way. Apply it on the blemish and blend it in by patting with your fingertips.

'If you like to wear foundation, apply that first and then put the concealer on over the foundation. This will give you plenty of cover for small veins, scars and under-eye shadows as well as spots and the skin discoloration they leave when they dry off. Use a light touch with both base and concealer . . . less always looks less obvious, and less like a cover up job.

'Always apply powder with a velour puff – the excess can be brushed off with a big brush and downward, outward sweeps to smooth it off and flatten fine facial hair. Powder helps to hold make-up much longer, and gives a more finished look. It's very important if your skin is oily or blemished because it makes scarring and distended pores less obvious.

'You can camouflage a multitude of minor skin faults with a light textured foundation, a little concealer and some powder. If spots are at the raised and bumpy stage, the bumps will still show of course, but it will disguise discoloration. I must emphasise that this treatment isn't for very bad outbreaks. These need medical attention and a lot of make-up won't help.

'Use the rest of your cosmetics to take attention away from the outbreak area. If the spots are on your forehead, choose a bright lipstick. If they're on your chin, make much of your eye make-up and play down your mouth with a neutral, brownish lip shade. So many girls with difficult skins hide under their hair, and have it hanging down around their faces with fringes flicking their eyelashes. Don't do this except perhaps for special occasions. If your face is oily, your hair's likely to be oily too and you're only adding to the grubbiness your face has to put up with from being out and about all day.

'There are three rules for a difficult skin and they are to be clean, be gentle and leave it alone. Wash morning and evening with a cleansing bar, or you can use a milk or lotion and follow with a gentle freshener – and use a moisturiser. Use an exfoliator twice or three times a week and do try to have a regular professional facial. A good beauty therapist does so much for skin and will advise you on how to look after it at home.

'Never poke at a spot yourself. I know we've all done it – caught a horrified glimpse in the mirror and felt compelled to squeeze. Resist the temptation. Squeezing risks passing bacteria around, and it can lead to scarring.

'I can't tell you how much I'm against fierce cleansers. If your skin's oily and spotty, they'll just aggravate the situation. When lotions carry boasts on what deep cleansers they are and how you'll see unbelievable amounts of deep down dirt just lifted away on your piece of cotton wool, what you're so often seeing is layers of your skin. Some of these cleansers and clarifiers are like paint stripper. They rip at the protective layer, and make your skin more sensitive and difficult, and they also harden it up.

'Do remember to look after your insides. One of the kindest things you can do for your skin is to drink water, I don't think you can ever have too much of it. It flushes the kidneys, gets rid of toxins and gets everything working better.'

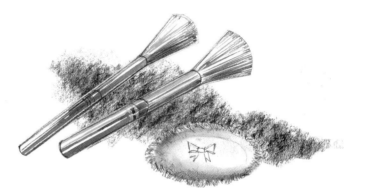

'Although men's skin tends to be coarser, it responds to treatments and products in exactly the same way as female skin. While the daily shave means that most male skins have the advantage of being exfoliated regularly during the beard removal process, men do tend to slap fierce after-shaves all over their faces. It's far better to use a moisturiser or an after-shave balm to soothe and calm the skin.

'Only a very small percentage of males use make-up, but there are two things that any man can do to look better without looking as though he's wearing cosmetics. The first is to wear concealer to disguise spots and blemishes. This should be chosen to match – as near as possible – the skin tone, and applied in exactly the same way as women would do, using a little brush and blending it in well with fingertips. Bronzers are a good idea if you want to look healthier and get rid of that washed-out look.

'The main criteria for men is that they don't look obvious, don't streak and don't come off or mark anything if they put their hand to their face, or someone else does. Powder bronzers look like make-up, and some gels are difficult to apply without streaking. I find the best formula is a cross

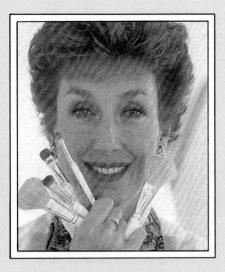

Left: Barbara Daly, well-known make-up artist and creator of Colourings.

1. Make up your face in a good, even light - avoid shadows and brilliant sunlight.

2. Apply foundation with a damp sponge to give you a 'professional' finish.

3. Concealer when applied with a fine brush and fingertips will disguise blemishes.

4. Loose powder will increase make-up's staying power, particularly if skin is oily.

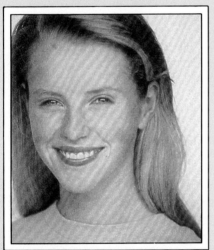

1.

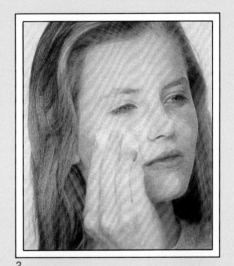

2.

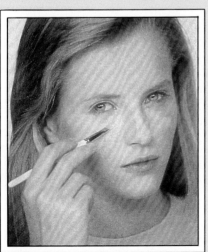

3.

4.

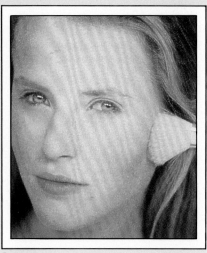

5.

5. Apply powder blusher after face powder. Use a large brush and a very light touch.

6. Eye shadow adds life to your eyes and takes attention away from any blemishes on the chin area.

7. Eye shadow and highlighter should be blended so there are no harsh edges.

8. Liptint adds gloss to a lipstick base - use it if your lips are well-shaped and youthful.

9. A day make-up should enhance your looks and conceal any flaws in your complexion.

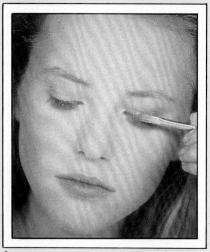

6.

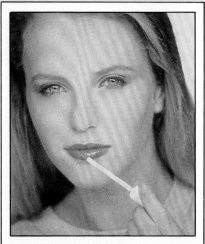

8.

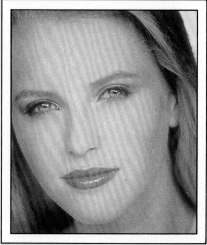

7.

9.

between a milk and a gel. Put a little in the palm of your hand and apply it from there. Make a final check under and around nostrils and eyebrows to see that there are no obvious traces lurking there.'

SKIN CAMOUFLAGE

You've no doubt heard someone say – or been known to say yourself – 'I can't possibly go out looking like this!' when *this* was a small crop of pimples that had left their mark, a bruise that would disappear within days or a temporary dose of dark shadows under the eyes. So, just imagine the distress and feelings of social isolation in someone with a *real* skin disfigurement, such as a massive birthmark, scar, disturbance in pigmentation or any major skin disorder.

When cosmetic surgery is not or is only partly the answer, there is a long wait for it to be done, treatment for something that will eventually get better is taking an age to work, or if there is any permanent skin disfigurement, cosmetic camouflage, using specially formulated covering creams, can quite literally make life worth living.

The creams are opaque and are designed to conceal discolorations and blemishes on all parts of the face and body. When applied properly to clean, dry skin, these products will last all day (but check if clothing is rubbing them), whatever the day holds. They are waterproof and won't disappear on sporting types who sweat profusely, plough up and down swimming baths or love watery activities of any sort. They contain filters to protect the skin from UV rays, and this is very important when pigment is lacking, or the sun has an adverse effect on the condition. There is a large choice of shades, so every possible skin colour is catered for and, of course, it is sometimes necessary to use several shades on one skin to even out the tone.

The creams are meant to be used sparingly – two thin layers may be better than one thicker one – and on large areas they may be applied with a sponge to obviate a flat, false look; a lip or eyeliner brush may be used in pits and folds. Powder seals the day-long finish. Ordinary foundation can be used over camouflage cosmetics if wished, and lip and eye make-up from a favourite cosmetic range. But, as the total success of the products depends on subtle and expert application, it's important initially to have the advice and practical help of a specially trained person who will show you exactly the colours needed and the best way to apply them. The products can be used on children and men. (A grey toner provides beard shadow where hair follicles have been damaged.)

Most camouflage cosmetics can be obtained from a chemist's shop and, in some cases, are available on prescription. The British Red Cross runs a marvellous Cosmetic Camouflage Service and has specially trained members attached to hospitals and clinics throughout the country. The dermatology unit of your hospital will give advice and explain the procedure for getting help (it is necessary to have a letter of referral from a GP, dermatologist, consultant or plastic surgeon) *or* you could contact the country branch headquarters *or* the National headquarters of the British Red Cross.

CHAPTER EIGHT

COSMETIC AND CORRECTIVE SURGERY

The late David Niven liked to tell this story of one of his social gaffes when he threw out this one-liner at a Hollywood dinner party, 'You could tell his surgeon from the cut of his face!' A glance around the table showed him he was sitting with a group of make-overs.

Britain isn't as cosmetically nip and tuck orientated as some countries, but has long been acknowledged as the home of experts at reconstructive and corrective surgery when genetic faults, illness or injury have destroyed or damaged skin, or nature has dealt a life-crippling blow in the shaping of some part of a face or body. It is perfectly possible too, to have first-class surgery to combat the effects of ageing or a feature about yourself that you hate, but isn't considered medically distressing. But it's more than likely that you'll have to pay all the costs in these cases.

When such an operation is considered, find out your real reasons for wanting it. For instance people often consider taking such steps when a relationship is on the rocks, but in fact no-one ever breaks up *just* because a nose is the wrong shape, breasts are too large or too small, or a face is looking a bit wrinkled. If you're convinced your reasons are sound, and it's right for you, shop around after getting advice from your doctor. Don't go to a clinic purely on the basis of an advertisement in a newspaper. Any good prospective surgeon will also question you about your motives and expectations, and look into your medical background and lifestyle.

Much 'cosmetic' surgery is impracticable for overweight people or those who indulge in large weight fluctuations. Sunbathers, smokers and people with a fairly high alcohol intake may not keep their new looks for long. You must be aware that there is likely to be discomfort and some risk if you are having an operation and anaesthetic. Costs can be high, too. Find out just how much is involved including stays in hospital and possible convalescence periods. Certainly no surgery should be undertaken without deeply considering the pros and cons. Someone very involved in the beauty business has remarked that having this type of surgery is rather like decorating a room in your home. Do up one area, and it shows how well-worn the rest looks.

FINDING A SURGEON

Plastic or aesthetic surgeons will require a letter of referral from a GP, dermatologist or consultant. If you are very reluctant to go to your family doctor for what you feel he or she might consider a 'vanity' request don't be put off. It is not unknown for some people to find their surgeon first, and the surgeon will then contact the GP. The surgeon should be a member of the British Association of Plastic Surgeons or the British Association of Aesthetic Plastic Surgeons – which means he holds or has held a consultant post in plastic surgery within the NHS. Personal recommendation is also a reassuring way to find your surgeon. If you know someone who has had treatment or surgery and is happy with the results, see if they will talk to you about it.

When you have made a preliminary choice, go for a discussion. You *must* be told about the drawbacks as well as the assets, the possible pain as well as the future pleasure. The consultation can take some time. No reputable surgeon will imply that if you are forty or fifty even a full face lift will make you look twenty again but it will make you look several years younger and *fitter*.

Look for someone who will discuss all the possibilities of minor surgery – peeling, collagen or fat implants, eyelid surgery – and will tell you how well this will work for you, or if it won't work well, why. It's a very good sign if surgeons are busy, you know that they are popular, and have had good results with their work.

Finally, you must feel that the person and the place are right for you. If you're in the least unhappy, move on.

A *plastic surgeon* deals primarily with disfigured or malformed bodies and faces caused by accidental or natural causes.

An *aesthetic surgeon* works on features and parts of the body that are not as good as they once were or are not as perfect as you would like them to be.

TREATMENTS AND SURGERY FOR THE FACE

SKIN PEELING

When the surface of the skin has been spoiled or scarred, whether shallowly or deeply, there are several methods of peeling which can correct or help the situation.

Exfoliation

Exfoliation with scrub creams or mechanical exfoliants plus time will do much for very shallow scars which have marked the skin's surface, but pitted scars need stronger methods.

Chemical peeling

Chemical peeling must be done by a doctor or dermatologist and involves the application of a caustic preparation which burns off the outer layers of skin. During the seven days or so following the treatment, the horny layer forms a crust which then peels revealing fresh, improved skin. There is some pain, swelling and discomfort during treatment and healing time. Sunlight and sunbathing should be shunned for six months or so after treatment to avoid the likelihood of pigmentation patching. Treatment can be repeated several months later if necessary. As well as removing superficial scarring, peeling can be used to improve skin texture or remove very fine surface lines. The possibility of pigmentation problems means this process is not suitable for very dark skins.

Dermabrasion

Dermabrasion goes slightly deeper than peeling and is rather like having a mini 'Black & Decker' working on your face. The epidermis is abraded with an electrically operated machine and brushes or a disc. Recovery time is longer than with peeling and it may take about three months for skin to look better than new. Again, sunshine can lead to pigmentation patching and should be avoided for several months and the treatment may not be suitable for dark skins. Dermabrasion must be done by an expert medical practitioner. It can be used to treat acne scars (when the acne is no longer active) and wrinkles.

COLLAGEN OR FAT IMPLANTS

These implants are a relatively simple, painless and foolproof way of filling in pitted scars and wrinkles. The process is also used to make fuller or shapelier lips. Liquid collagen (extracted from animal hide) is inserted into the area to be plumped up via a sterile needle and syringe. The collagen remains liquid for a few seconds to allow for manipulation in the case of lip re-shapes. It takes little time and needs only the application of an anaesthetising cream. There is little pain involved in the process and few problems (patch tests are done beforehand to test for allergy). The latest implants use fat from the clients own body instead of collagen. Like all good things, there are drawbacks:

1. It's not cheap, of course.

2. Your own body gradually absorbs the collagen, so results last only a year or so.

3. Injections of your own body fat can last indefinitely, but you must be prepared for some dying off of the implanted cells which means it may be necessary to have more than one treatment.

LID LIFTS *(Blepharoplasty)*

With age and/or genetic predisposition, the upper eyelid can become puffy or crêpey and bags can form under the eyes on lower lids. To remove them, cuts are made in the socket of the upper eyelid and just below the lashes of the lower lid and excess skin or fatty tissue is removed. These operations may be carried out under local anaesthetic and sedation. There is initial bruising and swelling and there may be a little discomfort for a few weeks. Scars are usually virtually invisible after a while. It is a very effective remover of obvious ageing characteristics and may be done where there is medical need on younger people. Margaret Thatcher's admission to having had this tidying up operation may help popularise it with people other than the show business fraternity.

NOSE *(rhinoplasty)*

Noses can be re-shaped to correct breathing difficulties, size (either too big or too small) and shape (crooked or broken). Surgery may be done under general anaesthetic or local anaesthetic plus sedation. The skin is lifted off the cartilage and bone and these can be made smaller, larger or re-modelled. The skin is then re-shaped over the understructure and all stitching is internal, so there are no visible scars (unless nostrils have been narrowed). There will be extensive bruising, swelling and discomfort for at least a week, and the nose may be tender for some time after it's looking good.

EARS *(otoplasty)*

Large and prominent ears have ruined many a child's school days, but as the ears are more or less fully-grown by the time a child is five or six, there is little need for this particular suffering. The operation to make them flatter is quite simple, and can be done under local anaesthetic. Scars are behind the ears and are virtually invisible. Incisions are made behind the ear, the excess cartilage is removed, and skin tightened and stitched. The major part of recovery is over in a week or so. (A bandage has to be worn during that time to keep them in their new place.)

FACELIFT *(rhytidectomy)*

Skin on the neck and cheeks is lifted and re-shaped over the bone structure, and excess skin is trimmed away. All stitching will be around the ears and hairline (and can easily be concealed by women – men may have more difficulty). This is an anti-ageing operation that will correct droopy jowls, nose to mouth lines, dropped mouths, scraggy necks and crow's feet (not eyelid droop or puffiness). Due to the length of operating time (about 3 hours) and the delicacy of the re-shaping (just the right amount of skin has to be taken away to make the patient look younger and healthier, but not so much that it produces a permanent 'rictus' grin) it's usually done under general anaesthetic. Normal living can be resumed in most cases after about three weeks, but discomfort will last much longer.

If ageing or other problems are localised, parts of the face may be operated upon – the upper face and brow, the neck and chin and the mid-face area.

CORRECTIVE SURGERY FOR THE BODY

BREASTS

Reduction

An over-large bust may lead to many problems, from too much ribald attention to backache and drawbacks when playing sport. During the operation breast tissue, fat and skin is removed and the nipple may be re-positioned which involves incisions (and therefore some scarring) under and around the breasts and around the nipple. The operation can take a couple of hours per breast under general anaesthetic. Life must be taken very gently for at least a month afterwards and reasonably gently for many more weeks after that. It is usually possible to breast feed after this operation, but of course, future pregnancies or a weight change can undo some of the benefits of the operation.

Enlargement

To make breasts larger or look more filled out, some form of gel or liquid filled implant is inserted, if possible from beneath the breasts, so scars are not obvious. Implants do not prevent future breast feeding and the reshaped breasts look and feel quite natural.

Again, this operation takes place under a general anaesthetic and vigorous movement is curbed for many weeks. If this operation follows a partial or radical mastectomy, skin grafts may be necessary and there may have to be several operations to complete the reconstruction process fully.

Drooping breasts can be lifted by the insertion of an implant (as in augmentation), if the droop isn't too severe. If breasts are very saggy and/or large they have to be re-shaped in an operation similar to breast reduction.

There has been controversy – particularly in the US – about the possible risks of some breast implants. In the UK all relevant bodies, including the government's Chief Medical Officer, have declared that there is no evidence to suggest that they are not safe. Breast implant operations continue to be done when necessary or desirable.

OTHER AREAS FOR IMPROVEMENT

It is possible to have excess tissue, fat and skin removed from the buttocks and abdomen. These processes can involve muscle tightening and are quite lengthy, painful and radical operations. Abdomen reconstruction leaves quite visible scars in the area. Chins can be made larger or reduced to improve the profile. Both these operations mean eating solids is difficult for many days afterwards.

LIPOSUCTION

Liposuction is a type of body sculpturing, that can be used when hips/thighs/buttocks are disproportionately large. Fat cells are aspirated by a surgeon using a sort of surgical vacuum cleaner. The process takes place under general anaesthetic, and demands an experienced surgeon who will remove the right amount of fat cells from the right areas to improve shape and to balance both sides of the body. Heavy bruising lasts for up to three weeks, but when this and any other swelling disappears, scars are small and virtually invisible. Results are best where skin elasticity is good, and subsequent effort must be made to keep or make the area firm. I have seen it work beautifully on a thirty-five year old who was subsequently inspired to follow sensible eating habits and a regular exercise routine.

It must be borne in mind that liposuction is *not* a treatment for the overweight and if fat will respond to a combination of diet and exercise, then they are the best ways to deal with it. Liposuction is for people who find that to reduce troublesome areas sufficiently, the rest of their body dwindles to near skin and bone.

'Heavy legs' are not the only area where liposuction can be used to re-shape the body successfully. Although the most common areas are buttocks, thighs, ankles and abdomen, it can be an ideal way to deal with double chins or even re-sculpt the face to some extent. In all cases, the surgeon will emphasise that maintaining ideal body weight and taking regular exercise is a vital part of the continuing success of this surgical treatment.

CHAPTER NINE

ALTERNATIVE THERAPIES

Watching television provides a good illustration of how the skin reacts almost instantly to the emotions and the workings of the mind. Those close-ups of the Wimbledon finalists, for instance, when one of them is points away from losing the match, show them looking lined, tense and old (even if they're very young). Then if the match goes their way, in the interview given only a short time later you'll see them looking young, athletic and glowing. You must have noticed, too, how much better you look when you've changed from an unrewarding job to a new and stimulating one, enjoying an exciting love affair or even when you've thrown yourself enthusiastically into a new hobby or interest.

When you're happy and well, skin colour and texture improve and (this is something you can see better on others than in the flat reflection of a mirrored image of yourself) the skin seems to be plumped out, and full of life. The way your skin works and looks can never be separated from the health of your body, mind and spirit. Most alternative therapists work on this premise, whether you're seeing them for a skin problem or for any other symptoms of a body that's out of balance. Alternative therapists treat the whole being rather than the disease or disorder.

So far, I've restrained myself from telling personal stories to push a point, but here's a break in the rule. Some years ago I had a totally debilitating illness, labelled as a virus by my very caring GP who arranged tests, prescribed plenty of rest and dished out no drugs. He soon sent me to see a specialist who found that there were lots of things wrong with my body, but he could only agree with the GP's diagnosis and gentle remedies.

After three months when I was no better and the quality of life had deteriorated to near zero, a friend recommended a traditional acupuncturist she knew. Within two visits I was virtually 'cured'. On my next appointment with the specialist he said 'God, you're better – what happened?' as I walked through the door. I hate to admit it now, but I hesitated before telling him of my visits to the acupuncturist. 'Brilliant', he said immediately, 'I was going to suggest something like that. I only wish I could afford to do the training myself.'

I'm telling this story principally to illustrate the fact that people who are trained in conventional medicine are increasingly acknowledging the possible benefits of alternative medicine and sometimes also practise it. Alternative therapists will invariably send a patient for orthodox medical investigation and treatment if they feel it necessary. Practitioners from both forms of medicine are occasionally joining forces.

While a full run-down on all the various types of alternative therapy would fill a book, here are a few that have remarkable results. In each case the whole person is treated rather than the disease or disorder, and they've all been proven to work well over a very long time.

ACUPUNCTURE

Acupuncture is part of the discipline of traditional Chinese medicine. First chronicled around four thousand years ago in China, it has been used in Europe for more than two hundred and fifty years. It is based on the concept that vital energy, or chi, has to flow freely along specific channels, called meridians, and body, mind and spirit must be balanced for everything to function satisfactorily. If there is a break or blockage in that flow, illness or less than total health will result.

Traditional acupuncture follows the classical Chinese perception of a person through the Chinese theory of the five elements. These elements are fire, earth, metal, water and wood, and each element relates to a group of organs and their widest possible function. The major organs (heart, lungs, kidney, liver etc) are connected through the meridians or lines of energy flow, and the acupuncture points situated along these meridians (as shown on traditional charts) will be used for treatments. Each of the five elements give out their own characteristic signals which indicate to the acupuncturist the state of that particular element and its relationship to the other elements. The acupuncturist will act upon the observations to get the patient's natural powers of recuperation to function better.

There are other systems of traditional acupuncture. For instance, one is based on the Chinese view of disorders of particular organs measured according to the eight principles (yin–yang, hot–cold, interior–exterior, deficiency–excess) and by consideration of the special characteristics of the internal organs, the channels and collaterals. Although these terms may be unfamiliar, and seem strange to Western sensibilities, they are part of a system of orderly diagnosis and treatment in another culture and, unless you are a great questioner, you will be largely unaware of all this during your treatment.

Initial sessions with a traditional acupuncturist may take up to two hours and will include close questioning (and listening) about your health, your lifestyle and how you respond to life in every way. Your pulses will be carefully taken. Your skin – its colour, tone, vitality, dryness, dampness, odour – is a key source of information to the acupuncturist. Touch and sight are as important as question and answer at every session. You should not wear make-up or perfume, have a heavy meal, drink strong coffee, alcohol, or have a hot bath before a session, as they can all interfere with diagnosis and treatment.

When the acupuncturist has made the diagnosis, and decided upon treatment, needles will be inserted at certain acupuncture points, and manipulated for a few seconds or swiftly removed (sometimes they can be retained for twenty minutes or so) in order to promote changes in the pattern of energy flow. You will not be stuck like a pin cushion (a very common misconception about acupuncture in people who have never experienced it). The practitioner will do the least possible work in order to help your body to heal itself. If you shy away from injections, it's important to know that the sensation is not at all similar. Acupuncture is virtually painless and feels rather like a fingernail resting on your skin with light pressure followed by a tiny 'grab' as the needle gets to the right spot of the meridian.

Acupuncture treatment can involve moxibustion – the burning of a small cone of Chinese herbs (Chinese mugwort) on the acupuncture point just until heat is felt – which is used to stimulate the energy flow. Some practitioners also use vacuum cups, which cling tightly to the acupuncture points and stimulate the flow of energy in the meridian. Occasionally, a mild electric current may be passed through the needles into the skin. This is a technique which is particularly appropriate for pain relief.

Traditional acupuncture may be used to help your body unravel from various states of ill-health, to make it stronger, or as a preventative treatment to help you maintain good health. Acupuncture is recognised by practitioners of orthodox Western medicine as being helpful for people who suffer from migraine, and some doctors trained in conventional medicine use a modified form of acupuncture to relieve pain in cases of back trouble, osteoarthritis, frozen joint syndrome etc. There is now experimental evidence which suggests that the stimulation of certain points releases forms of endorphin in the brain and spinal cord which modulate pain.

Traditional acupuncturists have to train for three to four years, so if you wish to find a properly qualified practitioner look for one who is registered. The Council of Acupuncture has a directory of British Acupuncturists which will be sent on request.

HERBAL MEDICINE AND CHINESE HERBS

Just as many animals have an uncanny instinct which leads them to eat certain plants when they are unwell, there's no doubt that humans have used plant life to nourish and heal their bodies since time immemorial, and many races living far from sources of conventional medicine have always had a successful pharmacy of plants around them to treat illness and injury. Herbal treatments are the oldest form of medicine known to man in all parts of the world. Writing came later, but use of herbal treatments and remedies were certainly chronicled more than 4000 years ago in China, and herbs were much used by the ancient Egyptians, Greeks, Romans and Anglo-Saxons. In the sixteenth, seventeenth and eighteenth centuries John Gerard, John Parkinson and Nicholas Culpeper published their still-famous works on herbal medicine in Great Britain.

In the past hundred years or so, scientists have discovered that many traditional herbal remedies contain chemical constituents which have a measurable activity in the body and many drugs much used in orthodox medicine come from plants. But, in the early nineteenth century, the practice of herbal medicine began to go into a decline in the Western world, partly because its practitioners weren't 'moving with the times', and partly because the new science of pharmacology reacted against the inexactitudes of herbal preparations and, perhaps, partly because there are fashions in everything, and people wanted the short, sharp 'cure' for a disease rather than the slower-working, gentler herbal remedies. In China, herbal medicine (and many other alternative therapies) have continued to be practised side by side with modern orthodox medicine.

A renewed interest in all things natural, the continuing success of herbal medicine for treating a variety of disorders, and the current disillusionment with modern drugs have served to reinstate plants as a popular source of health and well-being. Many toiletries and skin care products now boast of plant ingredients and orthodox medicine is re-examining the herbal roots of modern medicine and researching the benefits of the whole plant as opposed to simply isolating the active principles. It is now appreciated that other parts of plants although apparently pharmacologically inert, can still play a significant role. To give just one instance, meadowsweet is a good source of salicylic acid, the main constituent of aspirin. Isolated as a drug, this frequently causes stomach problems. Yet in herbal medicine, meadowsweet may be used to treat inflammation of the stomach, because its other constituents protect the stomach lining from the effect of the salicylates.

Herbal medicine is often successful in treating skin disorders over which, as yet, Western orthodox medicine has limited control and no cure. Such are the notable results of Chinese herbal medicine in this field that the National Eczema Society is helping to fund research into it by dermatologists at the Great Ormond Street Hospital for Sick Children.

Despite the difference in cultures, and the distance involved which proved almost impossible to overcome until comparatively recently, there is a very close link in much of the diagnosis, treatment and many of the remedies of Western and Chinese herbal medicine. The whole person is considered, rather than the disease or disorder.

Diagnosis includes a detailed case history, including questions about lifestyle, the study of the patient's appearance, appetite, temperature control, temperament, posture, tone of voice and particularly the appearance of the skin and tongue. Symptoms of a disorder, such as a fever, are not suppressed, but cooled or relaxed or warmed and stimulated according to the type of fever involved. Herbal antibiotics stimulate the body's own defences, and herbal tonics which supply vitamins and trace elements and encourage the elimination of waste materials are used when the body is weak in order to improve its own powers of recovery. Both fields of herbal medicine require the patient actively to participate with diet, exercise, relaxation techniques, deep breathing and, sometimes, the use of positive visualisation. Both ascribe different temperatures to herbs – hot, cold, warm, cool and neutral. Hot diseases must be cooled, and cold diseases must be warmed, so the remedy is taken from the force in nature which is related to the failing force within the body.

In Chinese herbal medicine, collecting information on the patient and making diagnosis is similar to acupuncture. Smell and touch (including pulse diagnosis) is taken into account as well as asking, looking and listening. Signs and symptoms are classified according to the eight principles and characteristics of the internal organs and channels to establish generally the location, temperature and strength of the disorder. The eight principles are yin and yang (which indicate the pattern of disharmony in the body), interior and exterior (to measure the depth of the disorder), deficiency and excess (the strength of the disorder versus the body's resistance), and cold and hot (the nature of the disorder).

The healing process seeks to achieve a balance between the Chinese concept of the five elements which are perceived as having their counterparts in the human body. This gives rise to the tastes by which medicinal plants are evaluated. Fire gives rise to bitterness and bitter tasting herbs drain and dry; earth gives rise to sweetness and sweet herbs tone up the body and may reduce pain; metal gives rise to acridity, and acrid herbs disperse; water gives rise to saltiness and salty herbs nourish the kidneys; wood gives rise to sourness and sour herbs nourish the body and prevent loss of body fluids and vital force. Bland herbs which have none of these tastes may have a diuretic effect.

Chinese medicine also evaluates food by taste and temperature. Therefore, someone with a 'cold' disease may be prescribed a diet of what Chinese traditional medicine terms warming foods, whereas someone with a 'hot' condition may be prescribed what they categorise as cooling foods.

Bad skin conditions, like any disorder or illness, are a sign that the body is not in harmony and that the vital organs are not functioning properly. Eczema conditions, for instance, will not be treated as 'just eczema'. If there are seeping blisters it will suggest an accumulation of body fluids, and the digestion may be treated to clear this problem, redness of the skin and tongue (fire) calls for cooling herbs, and chronic eczema can be treated with tonic herbs to cleanse and strengthen the Chi and blood, or the whole body.

Treatments are individual. There is certainly no standard formula. They may include special diets, ointments and a herbal medicine made up of a balanced mixture taken from a choice of many plants. As Michael McIntyre, acupuncturist and Chinese and Western herbalist says 'There is no special secret formula. So much depends on the diagnosis and individual prescription for the particular patient. It's like an expert tailor making a suit. Each prescription is made to measure rather than off the peg.'

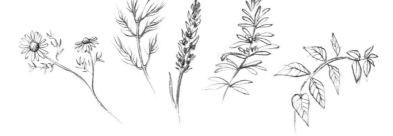

HOMOEOPATHY

Homoeopathy is a system of medicine based on the law of similars or 'like curing like'. Although the principle was known to the ancient Greeks, Dr Samuel Hahnemann developed it in the early nineteenth century. Appalled by the purging, blistering, blood-letting and other dangerous treatments of medicine at that time, he looked for a safe, gentle and effective alternative. By chance, he was experimenting with quinine (a known cure for malaria fevers) and found that a small dose given to his healthy body would produce symptoms of malaria. Testing drug after drug on himself and his followers, he found that extreme dilutions of drugs which in a healthy body produced certain symptoms, would cure sick people presenting similar symptoms. This extensive programme of drug testing with careful notes on all the symptoms experienced were called 'provings'. At the time of his death in 1843, Hahnemann had conducted provings on ninety-nine substances. Six hundred others were added to homoeopathic medicine by the beginning of the twentieth century, and the number is ever increasing.

Homoeopathic remedies are derived from animal, vegetable and mineral sources, and sometimes from diseased tissue, conventional drugs, allergens and cultures of bacteria. The minute doses, called 'potencies', are prepared by successive dilutions alternated with shakings which increase the curative properties and remove all poisonous or undesirable side effects.

If you know nothing about homoeopathic medicine, and find the concept strange, the same principle is used in allopathic (conventional) medicine for vaccines and innoculations.

The individual is very important in homoeopathic medicine with the physical, mental, emotional and environmental picture of the patient being matched by one of the drug pictures derived from the provings of remedies. One of the principles of homoeopathy is that people vary in response to an illness or disorder according to their basic temperament. A specific remedy is not automatically given for a specific disorder, the patient is treated rather than the disease. In the simplest terms a tall, thin person with a certain type of skin disorder, an equable temperament and a happy lifestyle, would not necessarily be given the same remedy as a short, fat person with a choleric temperament, even though the skin disorder might look the same.

Traditionally, only one preparation is given at a time because homoeopaths believe that the several symptoms which appear are part of one disorder. Symptoms are not suppressed, as it is believed they are a reflection of the body's fight to regain health, and stimulating them can encourage the body in its own healing process. The increase in symptoms for a short while proves to the homoeopath that he or she is on the right curative track.

While the remedy assists the patient back to health by stimulating nature's vital forces of recovery, appropriate diet, plenty of rest and congenial surroundings are helpful reinforcements to recovery. Patience is another part of the cure. This is essentially a natural healing system that helps the body back to harmony and well-being rather than delivering a very rapid 'cure'. Where a patient's vitality is low, the treatment may be long-term. For the same basic reason, homoeopathic treatments are very successful for babies and small children where natural vitality is high. Homoeopathy is practised as a safe alternative form of medical treatment in many countries throughout the world and, as the media has made much-known, is favoured highly by various members of the British Royal Family. There are GPs in many parts of the UK who provide homoeo-pathic treatment – within the NHS and privately – and several hospitals where homoeopathic treatment is available. (A letter of referral must be obtained from your GP.)

Homoeopathy is also effective in a wide range of veterinary problems, and there is a British Association of Homoeopathic Veterinary Surgeons.

NATUROPATHY

While Hippocrates is called the father of modern medicine there's little doubt that the healing methods of his day would have much more in common with herbal medicine and naturopathy. But naturopathy as an alternative system of medicine was developed and formalised in the mid to late nineteenth century in Germany and at the turn of this century in the United States and Great Britain.

As with many alternative therapies, naturopathy works on the concept that, given the right type of help, the body can heal itself and symptoms of a disease are part of the process of healing and should not be suppressed.

Whatever the symptoms of the disease or disorder, the entire body is treated. Naturopaths add nothing to the body, no drugs, herbs, potions, or needles, and treatment is based solely on natural external remedies, massage and changes of lifestyle that will help the body to heal and strengthen itself.

Consultations involve taking a detailed case history which includes the patient's physical and mental background and lifestyle. According to the diagnosis, there are a number of natural remedies that may be used on a particular patient. The composition and balance of diet is a fundamental part of treatment – for instance, naturopaths stressed the importance of eating the correct amount of fibre and fresh, raw fruits and vegetables for nearly a hundred years before it became an accepted part of modern dietary advice. Other treatments may include various appropriate forms of massage (many naturopaths are trained osteopaths), psychotherapy, acupressure and reflexology. One of the important features of naturopathy is that because treatment stems from the body itself, daily self-help is an intrinsic part of the treatment with suggested diet, suitable forms of exercise in the fresh air and hydrotherapy – using water at different temperatures and pressure to stimulate blood supply – becoming part of your new and healthier lifestyle.

While naturopaths use no drugs or treatments that will interfere with the body, they are increasingly working with psychotherapists, doctors, dermatologists and other specialists, and accept that certain orthodox medical treatments are beneficial (for instance the use of seaweed packs now much used in the treatment of conditions such as varicose ulcers).

Naturopathy is much used and has been successful in the treatment of acne, psoriasis, eczema and many inflamed skin conditions. As naturopath and osteopath, Jeremy Kenton, points out, 'If I shout at you, your skin will become pale or red. If you've had a hectic, stressful day your skin will be dry and flaky or grubby and greasy. If you are tired, your face will look drawn and pale. Skin is the first place to show any signs of emotion, fatigue and ill-health. With any skin disorder, there is always a predisposing internal cause which, given the right help or stimuli, your own body can help counteract.'

Naturopaths study full-time for four years and some may also be trained in allopathic (orthodox) medicine.

CHAPTER TEN

THE FUTURE OF SKIN CARE

Who would dare to forecast the future of skin care and corrective treatments fifty or even twenty years from now? Could we be gene-screening babies at birth to see if they are likely candidates for skin ailments (and other major potential defects) and pointing them towards a diet and lifestyle which will reduce their risk factors? Will plastic surgeons be able to transplant large pieces of human skin as they do vital, life-extending organs such as hearts, lungs or livers? Might often devastating skin disorders like eczema and psoriasis be as much a piece of history as scurvy? Is there a chance that we'll all be leaping around and wrinkle-free at seventy? Or will our cavalier attitude to our environment have zapped the ozone layer to the point when increasingly early signs of ageing and skin cancers are a new plague for the world's population?

Perhaps a touch of consideration towards the environment, a degree of DIY commonsense in the way we treat our own protective covering, and a modicum of social awareness and hand-in-pocket generosity directed ostensibly towards people with skin disorders and disfigurements, may help to provide the best chance for everyone's skin. In the meantime, what's the prognosis for the near future? People are living longer and not wanting to broadcast their chronological age by looks or attitude, yet too many of us are still conducting a love affair with the sun and equating baking a white skin to a thick brown crust with 'beautiful', a situation which all those involved in work on skin are aiming to change.

There is now tangible hope for people suffering from skin disorders and diseases with innovative research on cell and skin cell cultures, and increasing co-operation between orthodox Western and alternative medicine in the war against eczema and psoriasis. Cosmetic surgery and treatments are tipped as becoming much more commonplace (and not only by cosmetic surgeons). Skin care products will be formulated increasingly to protect our skins from irritants including all the sun's rays and to keep them blemish-free and looking young. And if you're bothered and bewildered by countless cosmetic display areas and batteries of potions and lotions that may or may not do some good for your skin, simplification and more constructive service at point of sale is an encouraging trend. Let's get some expert views on the future of skin care research and treatments.

COSMETICS

Diane Miles, pharmacist and Marketing Manager for Christian Dior predicts:

'In the UK nearly fifty per cent of women are over forty and there's an even higher percentage in some Western countries, so the future of skin care product research has to be with arresting the ageing process. There'll be further work into preventing the detrimental effects of the sun with screens and moisturisers incorporating substances to combat UVA, UVB, UVC and Infra-Red rays.

'The past five years have introduced moisturisers with increased powers of penetration and this will further improve with new moisturising materials and increased stability of carriers. Just as aspirin now have a wax coating on the tablet which allows for the slow and regular release of the drug resulting in better affinity with the body and fewer side effects, this indicates what we're doing and will increasingly be doing in the cosmetics industry.

'In our own brand we're working specifically for the more mature woman to help overcome the changes which occur suddenly in the skin at a certain time in a woman's life.

'I'm sure that the major skin care and cosmetic companies will move to more customer specificity. There will still be a wide selection, but choice will be simpler with, for example, one brand hypoallergenic, one natural, one for specific skin care needs, and more and more major brands will be offering a special service to the customer, such as facials at point of sale, computer read-outs, and skin scanners.'

DERMATOLOGY

David Fenton, Senior Registrar at the Dowling Skin Unit, at St Thomas' Hospital in London, agrees that the cosmetics houses will move towards greater simplification with ingredients kept to a minimum to reduce the risk of allergic reaction.

His view is, 'All that most skin needs is a good cleanser, and a moisturiser when and where necessary to make the skin less dry and stop irritants getting to it and moisture getting out. A simple moisturiser – preferably non-comedogenic – and a sunscreen during the day should be enough for most skins. Even if products contain ingredients that give them a higher potential for penetration of the top layers of skin, they may not work better than ordinary moisturisers. In addition, people *must* become more sensible about the damaging effects of the sun, particularly on pale Celtic skins and children's skins. Sun damage is not reversible. It may not be obvious for some years, but once it has happened, you can only prevent further damage. Appearance is very important to people's health and happiness and as we're all living longer, it is ridiculous to encourage premature ageing and put skins at high risk.'

CHANGING LOOKS

Cosmetic surgeon, Dr Alan Kingdon, Director of the Harley Medical Group points out that more of us are already following America's lead in taking stringent steps to look better and correct the more obvious signs of ageing.

'People will become more open about cosmetic surgery, they'll discuss what they've had done, and treat it like a visit to the dentist, as just another way of retaining youthful characteristics. People are already better informed on the subject. They know what's involved before they come to us to discuss treatment or surgery – which couldn't be said four or five years ago.

I feel that the future lies in many more people having minor surgery or treatments to offset the effects of ageing – eyelid surgery, liposuction, fat or collagen implants – rather than radical surgery.'

ECZEMA – EAST-WEST COLLABORATION

Anyone who suffers from eczema, or who has someone in the family with this skin disorder that can make life a constant misery, will be delighted to hear of the collaboration between a research team from the dermatology department at Great Ormond Street Hospital for Sick Children in London and a London-based Chinese doctor who is doing some dramatically effective work on severe eczema cases using traditional Chinese herbal remedies and treatment. To get the same effect, Western medicine would have to use strong drugs with possible side effects, yet Chinese herbal medicine appears to have none.

David Atherton, consultant in paediatric dermatology at Great Ormond Street, explains, 'We're very aware that our present treatment is just not adequate. We can help a good proportion of patients, but we're just not able to do something for every case. We're studying the use of Chinese herbal medicine for the treatment of eczema. Once we've learned more we could make it more widely available to our patients. Herbal treatments might be brought into Western medicine with GPs being able to prescribe them for a skin disease like eczema.'

BURN SURGERY

While heart, lung, liver and kidney transplants are carried out with a high degree of success, skin proves to be a trickier organ – a body likes its own skin. In bad burn cases, the glowing enthusiasm for 'wrapping' (to keep tissue fluids in and infection out) with laboratory-grown sheets of epidermis has lapsed. The laboratory grown epidermis didn't behave like ordinary skin. It didn't sweat, had little resistance to infection and couldn't be relied on to last long enough to allow the patient's own underlying skin to heal.

The latest techniques for dealing with patients with extensive burns (where own-skin grafts would mean more large and painful wounds for the patient) is explained by Tim Goodacre, Consultant Plastic Surgeon at the Radcliffe Infirmary, Oxford:

'We make a type of sandwich with a widely expanded mesh of the patient's own skin covered with a less widely expanded mesh of donor skin, usually that of a relative. Due to the Aids issue, we can no longer take anonymously donated skin. The patient's own expanded area of skin will have holes in it which will gradually fill in as it heals. The strong hope for the future is that cyclosporin – the immuno suppression drug used in heart and liver transplant surgery – will increasingly be brought into use to help prevent rejection of grafted donor skin.'

RESEARCH AND SKIN PROBLEMS

The ability to grow reconstructed human skin (RHS) – layered skin with a dermis and epidermis – in laboratory dishes has opened up infinite opportunities for research and experiment. Given the right nutritious mix and conditions, dermal cells added to a solution of jellified collagen develop into a small piece of dermis. A matchhead-sized piece of epidermis planted in this dermal mixture will grow in about three weeks to cover the dermis and make a small piece of multi-layered skin. Though lacking pigment, blood supply, hair follicles, sweat and sebaceous glands, RHS has been used in France for grafting purposes.

The ability to culture cells and skin cells in the laboratory provides a sophisticated and valuable tool for such varied research as studying the skin ageing process, studying and monitoring treatment in a variety of skin disorders and diseases (malignant melanoma, a virulent skin cancer, has been grown in RHS at London's Westminster Hospital, so it's possible to study growth and ways of curtailing that growth) and it will reduce the need for many animal experiments. The technique was pioneered in the UK (previously it was only available in France and the States) by a research team at the Westminster Hospital and is supported by a charity called the Skin Treatment and Research Trust (START).

Heading the Westminster Hospital team, consultant dermatologist Richard Staughton says: 'We have cultivated bits of dermis and dermal cells and used them to study how the fibroblasts work; the action of chemical messengers between the layers; the significant differences between psoriatic and non-psoriatic skin; to look at treatments of the body which may affect the skin; to monitor the treatment of cancer.

'Currently we're hoping to develop a diagnostic test for skin cancer by analysing chemical changes in the patient's urine; looking for information on eczema by studying the blood platelets; making skin biopsies of psoriatic HIV patients to find out if we can cast more light on psoriasis in HIV and non-HIV patients.'

ANIMAL EXPERIMENTS

Does the idea of all animal experiments drive you into a cold fury? Or do you fall into the great group who can tolerate the concept of their necessity for medical research, but curl up at the idea of animals enduring a lifetime of suffering so that you can safely pat on a new skin cream, put on your cosmetics or even shampoo your hair without the foam injuring your eyes.

The consumer surge towards cosmetics and toiletries heralded as 'cruelty-free' shows the strength of feeling about animal testing, certainly in the realms of what might be termed 'vanity' products. Let's remove some of the confusion and indeed hype from the subject and look at a rational and constructive approach.

FRAME (Fund for the Replacement of Animals in Medical Experiments) seeks to promote a moderate, but very determined answer to the question of all experiments on living animals, recognising that their immediate abolition is not possible if medical research is to continue seeking cures for human and animal diseases and new consumer products, drugs, industrial and agricultural chemicals are to be developed.

FRAME's stance is evolutionary rather than revolutionary. While their ultimate aim is to eliminate the need for live animal experiments, their immediate one is the development, validation and international promotion of replacement alternative testing methods. Where animal involvement can at present be justified, they work to minimise any suffering, pain or distress. In fact, alternative eye and skin tests are now at an advanced stage of development and validation and FRAME co-ordinates an ambitious research programme to investigate the potential of tissue culture as an alternative means of toxicity testing. Surrey and Nottingham Universities are working with them on skin cell cultures, seeing how they will respond to chemicals, then they'll be moving on to cosmetics, sunscreens and anti-ageing creams.

Dr Julia Fentem, Scientific Liaison Officer at FRAME gives their very balanced view on this emotive subject. 'We would like to be able to say "No animal testing", but at the moment without fully validated alternatives this could jeopardise consumer safety. It must be remembered that even when it comes to the production of something as potentially repetitive as a shampoo, the workforce exposed to products on an industrial scale may be subjected to high concentrations. The health and safety of the manufacturer, supplier and the environment must be protected as well as that of the consumer. And while you might feel no animal should suffer for your face, how would you feel if your child tried to make a meal of your moisturiser and became seriously ill?

'Many of the products in the cosmetics and toiletries category are for personal hygiene as well as prettification, and in some cases cosmetics can provide a means of facing the world with a degree of confidence when people have been born with severe blemishes or have suffered accidental or surgical scars. Whether they're considered unnecessary fripperies or essential items, the chemical ingredients of all cosmetics and toiletries have had to be tested for potential toxic effects by law which in the past has often meant the use of animal tests.

'However, in the UK, if the new formulations use previously screened ingredients, the new product need not be tested. The product which comes to you with claims such as "not tested on animals" is likely to contain ingredients which have been tested on animals at some time – although perhaps not in the past five years. Having said that, the number of animal experiments these days involving cosmetics is a fraction of a percentage of the total and has been falling consistently in recent years. Very few decorative cosmetics, such as eyeshadows and lipsticks, need to be tested these days. Cosmetic tests are also most readily open to replacement by alternative tests and the cosmetic industry has made a very large commitment to the search for alternatives both in its own research and developments and by supporting academic research and charities such as FRAME. Our goal is to develop methods for use in toxicity tests and safety assessment which will be so relevant that no animal testing will be needed.'

FRAME sponsors and conducts research into alternatives to animal-testing, working with research groups at Universities and Polytechnics. They are involved in a number of validation trials and are liaising with industrial companies in the UK and abroad. To avoid unnecessary repetition of animal tests they have established a data bank to provide scientists world-wide with up-to-date information on alternative methods in toxicology. They campaign and distribute information through a quarterly scientific journal, ATLA (Alternatives to Laboratory Animals) and a quarterly newsletter, FRAME NEWS, aimed at scientists, politicians, supporters and members of the general public. They maintain contact with sympathetic members of parliament through the All-Party Parliamentary Frame Group and provide balanced and informative educational material to schools and colleges.

Funds for research are obtained as specific donations from industrial companies, other charitable organisations, the EC and the Government. Parliamentary monitoring, education, publications, administration and FRAME's information services on alternatives rely on the generosity of other charitable trusts and the general public.

BIBLIOGRAPHY

Acne Morphogenesis and Treatment by Gerd Plewig and Albert M. Kligman, Springer-Verlag.

Alexander Technique, The by Liz Hodgkinson, Piatkus Books, 1988

Allergy – The Facts by Robert Davies and Susan Ollier, Oxford University Press, 1989

Alternative Therapy, BMA Publications, 1986

Beauty and Medicine by Robert Aron Brunetiere, Jonathan Cape, 1978

Beauty Treatment Handbook, The by Linda Zeff, Piatkus Books, 1988

Care of the Skin by Audrey Githa Goldberg, Heinemann Professional Publishing, 1988

Common Skin Problems by G. Colver and J.A. Savin, BMA Publications, 1988

Dictionary of Vitamins, The by Leonard Mervyn, Thorsons, 1984

Dr Fulton's Step-by-Step Program for Clearing Acne by James E. Fulton and Elizabeth Black, Barnes & Noble, 1984

Evening Primrose Oil by Judy Graham, Thorsons, 1988

Healing Plants by William A.R. Thomson (Ed.), Macmillan, 1980

Herbal Medicine for Everyone by Michael McIntyre, Penguin Books, 1988

Homeopathic Medicine at Home by Maesimund B. Panos and Jane Heimlich, Corgi Books, 1986

Illustrated Herbal, The by Philippa Back, Hamlyn, 1987

Les Nouvelles Esthetiques (various issues)

Skin Book, The by Arnold W. Klein, James H. Sternberg and Paul Bernstein, Sheldon Press, 1984

Taking Care of Your Skin by Dr Vernon Coleman, Sheldon Press, 1984

Using Essential Oils for Health and Beauty by Daniele Ryman, Century Hutchinson, 1986

Vogue Beauty and Health Encyclopedia by Christina Probert, Octopus, 1986

Your Skin and How to Live In It by Jerome Z. Litt, Ballantine Books, 1982

USEFUL ADDRESSES *(when writing please enclose SAE)*

Acne Support Group, 16 Dufour's Place, Broadwick Street, London W1V 1FE

To locate a qualified beauty therapist in your area:

BABTAC (British Association of Beauty Therapy and Cosmetology), 2nd floor, 34 Imperial Square, Cheltenham, Gloucestershire GL50 1QZ (tel 0242 570284)

To find a qualified aromatherapist contact one of the addresses below:

The Institute of Clinical Aromatherapy, 22 Bromley Road, London SE6 2TP

The International Federation of Aromatherapists, Department of Continuing Education, The Royal Masonic Hospital, Raven's Court Park, London W6 0TN (please send £1.40 for the directory of aromatherapists)

Tisser and Aromatherapy Institute, 65 Church Road, Hove, East Sussex BN3 2BD

BABTAC (address above)

To locate a qualified electrolysist contact one of the addresses below:

Margaret Anderson, British Association of Electrolysists, 18 Stokes End, Haddenham, Buckinghamshire HP17 8DX

Edna Derbyshire, The Institute of Electrolysis, Lansdowne House, 251 Seymour Grove, Manchester M16 0DS

To find an electrolysist using the Digital Blend System, contact:

The Hairdressing & Beauty Equipment Centre, Antonia House, 262 Holloway Road, London N7 6NE (tel 071–607 7475)

For advice and practical help with all aspects of skincare and make-up:

Joan Price's Face Place, 33 Cadogan Place, London SW3 2PP (tel 071–589 9062)

Face Facts, 73 Wigmore Street, London W1H 9LH (tel 071–935 8478)

Shahnaz Herbal, 5A Bathurst Street, London W2 2SD (tel 071–724 0440) Beauty therapists specialising in body and skin treatments, including threading, for Asian and non-Asian skin.

Flori Roberts and Dermablend Clinic, 158 Notting Hill Gate, London W11 3GQ (tel 071–229 4224)
Corrective and camouflage cosmetics for all skins. Skin care and cosmetics for black skin. Will give free advice and practical help to all clients. Also will provide details of stockists and mail order.

Cosmetic Camouflage Service, British Red Cross, 9 Grosvenor Crescent, London SW1X 7EJ (tel 071–235 5454)

Katherine Corbett, SRN, Upper Floor, 21 South Molton Street, London W1Y 1DD (tel 071–629 2210)
Specialist in the removal of minor skin care blemishes. Free skin care advisory service.

The National Eczema Society, 4 Tavistock Place, London WC1H 9RA (tel 071–388 4097)

The Psoriasis Association, 7 Milton Street, Northampton NN2 7JG (tel 0604 711129)

Society of Teachers of the Alexander Technique, 20 London House, 266 Fulham Road, London SW10 9EL (tel 071–351 0828)
For information and a list of qualified teachers.

The Council for Acupuncture, 179 Gloucester Place, London NW1 6DX (tel 071–724 5756)
For advice on acupuncture, a qualified acupuncturist in your area or a directory of British acupuncturists (please send an A5 SAE and £2 for the directory)

Register of Practitioners of Chinese Herbal Medicine, 21 Warbeck Road, London W12 8NS (please send an A5 SAE and £2 for the directory)

The British Homeopathic Association, 27A Devonshire Street, London W1N 1RJ

General Council and Register of Naturopaths, Frazer House, 6 Netherall Gardens, London NW3 5RR
To obtain the register of qualified naturopaths.

START (The Skin Treatment and Research Trust), Westminster Hospital, London SW1
To find out more about START and its fundraising activities.

FRAME (Fund for the Replacement of Animals in Medical Experiments), Eastgate House, 34 Stoney Street, Nottingham NG1 1NB (tel 0602–584740)
For further information about their aims and activities.

INDEX